Advanced Internal Family Systems for Therapists

Healing Complex Trauma, Dissociation, and Addiction

Candace Brett Parrish

Copyright © 2025 by Candace Brett Parrish All rights reserved.

No part of this publication may be reproduced, distributed, or transmitted in any form or by any means, including photocopying, recording, or other electronic or mechanical methods, without the prior written permission of the publisher or author, except in the case of brief quotations embodied in critical reviews and certain other noncommercial uses permitted by copyright law.

This book is intended for informational and educational purposes only for mental health professionals. It is not a substitute for professional clinical training, supervision, or consultation. The content herein is designed to offer advanced perspectives and techniques within the Internal Family Systems model. Readers are advised to use their professional judgment and adhere to ethical guidelines and scope of practice in their respective fields.

The names and scenarios depicted in this book are purely for illustrative purposes only. Any resemblance to actual persons, living or dead, or actual events is purely coincidental.

ISBN: 978-1-7641941-2-9

Isohan Publishing

Table of Contents

Chapter 1: Advanced IFS Concepts 1
Chapter 2: Advanced Techniques for Deepening the IFS Process 12
Chapter 3: IFS in Complex Trauma and Dissociative Disorders 31
Chapter 4: IFS in Addiction Treatment 40
Chapter 5: IFS Integration with Other Advanced Modalities 45
Chapter 6: Getting Through Tricky Client Situations 63
Chapter 7: Ethics and Growing as a Professional 71
Chapter 8: The Current State of Research and New Directions 78
Chapter 9: A Call for More Research and Professional Growth 86
References 90

Chapter 1: Advanced IFS Concepts

Imagine for a moment that your mind is not a single, unified entity, but rather a bustling inner community, much like a family. Each member of this internal family has its own thoughts, feelings, and ways of trying to help you. This is the heart of the Internal Family Systems (IFS) model, a way of understanding the human psyche that sees us as naturally made up of many parts, all guided by a wise and undamaged core Self.[1] While you might already know the basics of Managers, Firefighters, and Exiles, working with complex cases means looking much closer at these inner workings. It means seeing the subtle connections and hidden intentions that shape a person's inner world.

Nuances of Multiplicity: Beyond Basic Parts

In the early stages of learning IFS, we get to know the main players: Managers, Firefighters, and Exiles. Managers are like the planners and organizers of your inner world; they try to keep things running smoothly and prevent pain by being perfect, making plans, or taking care of others.[2] Firefighters are the quick responders, jumping into action when pain becomes too much. They might use things like substance use, self-harm, or avoiding situations to try and put out emotional fires.[2] And then there are the Exiles, the parts that hold onto deep emotional pain, beliefs, and memories from past hurts, often pushed away so you do not have to feel them.[2]

But here is where advanced IFS truly shines: the idea that there are **no bad parts**.[6] This is not just a nice thought; it is a powerful truth when you are working with people who have extreme or seemingly destructive parts. Think about parts that drive thoughts of ending one's life, severe addictions, or self-harm. It can feel scary to approach these parts. Yet, in advanced IFS, you learn to meet them with genuine curiosity and deep caring. You see that even these extreme parts are trying to help, even if their methods are misguided and cause more problems.[6]

This way of looking at things changes everything. Instead of just naming a part, you seek to understand its positive purpose. This non-judgmental view is key to building trust and safety inside a person's system. When parts feel truly seen and understood, they can relax their guard and begin to let go of their heavy burdens.[6] Your ability as a therapist to hold this kind, accepting stance, even when faced with very intense or frightening material, is a sign of advanced IFS practice. It shows you can be a steady, calm presence for your client, helping them feel safe enough to heal.

Let us look at some examples to make this clearer:

Case Example 1: The Overworked Perfectionist

Sarah, a 42-year-old marketing executive, came to therapy feeling completely burned out. She worked 70-hour weeks, constantly worried about making mistakes, and found it impossible to relax. She described an "inner critic" that pushed her relentlessly, telling her she was not good enough unless everything was perfect. In earlier therapy, she had tried to silence this critic, but it only seemed to get louder.

Using advanced IFS, her therapist helped Sarah understand that this "inner critic" was not trying to hurt her. Instead, it was a Manager part, working overtime to protect her from a deep fear of failure and rejection that an Exile part carried from childhood experiences. This Manager believed that if

Sarah was not perfect, she would be abandoned, just like she felt as a child. The therapist helped Sarah approach this Manager with curiosity, asking, "What are you trying to prevent from happening?" and "What are you afraid would happen if you stopped pushing so hard?".[6] As Sarah's Self connected with this Manager, it softened, realizing its extreme efforts were actually making Sarah miserable. It began to trust that Sarah's Self could handle any perceived failures, allowing it to relax its grip and find a less exhausting way to protect.

Case Example 2: The Secret Drinker

Mark, a 35-year-old father, struggled with a hidden drinking problem. He would drink heavily alone at night, feeling immense shame the next day. He felt like a failure and hated this part of himself. He had tried to stop many times, but the urge always returned, especially after stressful days at work or arguments with his wife.

His therapist, using the "no bad parts" lens, helped Mark see his drinking not as a moral failing, but as a Firefighter part trying desperately to help him.[6] This Firefighter would jump in to numb the overwhelming feelings of inadequacy and loneliness that an Exile part held. Mark's therapist asked the Firefighter, "What are you trying to do for Mark when he drinks?" The Firefighter revealed it was trying to make the pain go away, to help Mark relax, and to escape the heavy burden of feeling like he was not enough. By acknowledging the Firefighter's positive intent, Mark's shame lessened, and he could approach this part with compassion. This allowed the Firefighter to step back enough for Mark to connect with the lonely Exile, beginning the process of healing its pain rather than just numbing it.[6]

Case Example 3: The Self-Harm Protector

Chloe, a 19-year-old college student, had a history of self-harm when feeling overwhelmed by emotions. She felt a strong urge to cut herself when anxiety or sadness became too intense, describing it as a way to "feel something" or "release the pressure." She felt disgusted with herself afterward and kept it a secret.

Her therapist approached Chloe's self-harming part with deep respect and curiosity, understanding it as an extreme Firefighter trying to cope with unbearable emotional pain.[10] Instead of immediately trying to stop the behavior, the therapist asked, "What is this part trying to do for you when you cut?" The part communicated that it was trying to help Chloe survive, to distract her from emotional agony, and to give her a sense of control when everything else felt out of control.[10] This compassionate inquiry helped Chloe feel less alone and less judged. As the self-harming part felt understood and its positive intention acknowledged, it became willing to consider other ways to help Chloe, opening the door for healing the underlying Exiles that carried the intense emotional burdens.[10]

The Indestructible Self: Expanding the 8 Cs

At the very core of every person is the Self, a wise and undamaged essence.[1] Think of it as your true north, always present, always knowing how to heal. This Self is not something you have to build or create; it is already there, waiting to be accessed.[10] It shows up through eight special qualities, often called the 8 Cs:

Confidence, Calm, Compassion, Courage, Creativity, Clarity, Curiosity, and Connectedness.[1]

In complex situations, a person's access to their Self might be hidden by the strong actions of protective parts.[4] It is like the sun always being in the sky, but sometimes clouds (our parts) cover it up.[17] Advanced IFS practice is not just about helping people find their Self; it is about helping them live from this core place, even when things are tough inside.[16]

A really important point for therapists is telling the difference between true Self-energy and what we call "Self-like parts" (SLPs).[16] SLPs might seem like the Self because they show some of the 8 Cs, like being calm or compassionate. But they are still mixed with a protective agenda, often driven by fear or a need to control things.[16] For example, a "calm" SLP might be calm because it is trying to avoid conflict, not because it is truly at peace.

For you, as a therapist, recognizing and separating your own SLPs from your true Self-energy is super important.[16] You might have an "overly helpful therapist part" or a "caregiving part" that wants to fix or rescue your client. If you are blended with these parts, you might accidentally get in the way of your client's own healing.[16] When you work from your true, unblended Self, you become a steady, safe anchor for your client's system. This allows for deeper healing and change that might otherwise be blocked by your own unconscious reactions.[16]

Let us look at some examples of how this plays out:

Case Example 1: The Therapist's "Fix-It" Part

Dr. Evans, an experienced therapist, found herself feeling frustrated with a client, David, who seemed stuck in a cycle of self-sabotage. David would make progress, then suddenly pull back, missing appointments or dismissing insights. Dr.

Evans noticed a strong urge to "fix" David, to push him harder, and felt a sense of personal failure when he did not improve quickly.

Through her own supervision, Dr. Evans realized she was blended with a "Fix-It" SLP. This part, while well-meaning, was driven by a fear of not being a good enough therapist and a need to control the outcome. It mimicked Self-qualities like "courage" (to confront David) but was not truly coming from a place of open curiosity. Once Dr. Evans unblended from this SLP, she could approach David with genuine Self-compassion and curiosity. She realized David's "resistance" was a protective part, and her "Fix-It" part was actually making his protector work harder. From her unblended Self, she could calmly ask David's protector what it was afraid of, creating a space for true dialogue and progress.

Case Example 2: The Client's "Spiritual Bypass" SLP

Maria, a client working on childhood trauma, often spoke about "just letting go" and "being positive," even when discussing painful memories. She seemed calm and accepting, but her therapist noticed a lack of genuine emotion and a quick shift away from any discomfort. Maria's therapist wondered if this was true Self-energy or a protective pattern.

The therapist gently explored this with Maria, asking, "When you say 'just let go,' what part of you is saying that? Does it feel like your whole Self, or is there a part that wants to avoid the pain?" Maria connected with a "Spiritual Bypass" SLP, a part that had learned to use spiritual concepts to avoid feeling difficult emotions. This part was trying to protect a deeply wounded Exile that carried intense shame. While it appeared calm and wise, it was still a protector. By helping Maria differentiate this SLP from her true Self, Maria could then, from her Self, offer genuine compassion to the shame-filled Exile, allowing for real healing instead of just avoidance.

Case Example 3: The Leader's "Confident Performer" SLP

John, a CEO, presented as highly confident and decisive. He rarely showed vulnerability and always had a solution. His team, however, felt intimidated and disconnected. John's therapist noticed that while John appeared confident, there was a subtle rigidity and a fear of making mistakes underneath.

The therapist helped John explore his "Confident Performer" SLP. This part had developed early in his career to protect a younger, insecure Exile that feared being seen as weak. This SLP mimicked true Self-confidence but was actually driven by a need for external validation and control. When John connected with his true Self, he could see how this SLP, while helping him succeed, also kept him isolated. From his Self, John began to show more genuine vulnerability and compassion to his team, which fostered deeper trust and connection, something his "Confident Performer" part could not achieve on its own.[21]

Understanding Burdens: Personal and Legacy

In IFS, "burdens" are the painful emotions, beliefs, or memories that parts carry because of tough experiences.[3] Think of it like a heavy backpack that a part has been carrying for a long time. In advanced IFS, we learn that these burdens come in two main types, and understanding the difference can really change how you help someone heal:

- **Personal Burdens:** These are the negative thoughts, feelings, and body sensations that come directly from a person's own hurtful experiences.[22] For example, a part might carry the belief, "I am worthless," because of being neglected as a child.[4] This is a direct result of something that happened to them.

- **Legacy Burdens:** These are negative thoughts, feelings, and body sensations that have been passed down through generations, like from ancestors, or absorbed from big cultural or historical traumas.[22] A person might say something like, "This fear has always been in our family," or "My grandmother always said we had to be strong, no matter what." This points to a legacy burden, not something they experienced directly, but something they inherited or absorbed from their family or culture.[22]

Seeing legacy burdens adds a really important layer to advanced IFS work, especially when you are helping people with intergenerational trauma or cultural issues. It means that healing can go beyond just what happened in one person's life; it can also touch on experiences from their family history and wider community.[22] When legacy burdens show up, you might even think about bringing in other ways of working, like EMDR (Eye Movement Desensitization and Reprocessing) protocols that are designed for legacy issues.[22] This shows how IFS can work smoothly with other trauma-focused therapies to help with deep, long-standing patterns of suffering that have been passed down. This deeper understanding of burdens helps you offer more complete and culturally sensitive healing.

Here are some examples to illustrate these different kinds of burdens:

Case Example 1: The Burden of "Never Enough"

David, a 38-year-old artist, struggled with constant feelings of not being good enough, despite his artistic talent. He felt a deep sense of shame about his work, always believing it was flawed. He traced this back to his strict father, who rarely praised him and often pointed out his mistakes.

In therapy, David identified an Exile part that carried the burden of "I am fundamentally flawed." This was a **personal burden** [22], directly linked to his childhood experiences with his father. The therapist helped David's Self witness this Exile's pain and the belief it held. Through the unburdening process, David was able to release this heavy feeling, realizing it was a belief his child-part had taken on, not an actual truth about him. His Self could then offer comfort and acceptance to this part, allowing it to transform and bring its natural creativity forward without the weight of shame.

Case Example 2: The Burden of "Always Be Strong"

Maria, a 55-year-old woman, found it almost impossible to ask for help, even when she was struggling. She felt a strong internal pressure to "always be strong" and handle everything on her own. When she felt vulnerable, a part would tell her, "Don't be weak, no one will help you anyway." She could not pinpoint a specific event in her own life that caused this, but she remembered her grandmother, a survivor of a difficult historical period, often saying, "We must always be strong; there is no room for weakness."

Maria's therapist recognized this as a potential **legacy burden**.[22] The "Always Be Strong" part was carrying a belief passed down from her grandmother's generation, a survival strategy from a time when showing vulnerability could be dangerous. This was not Maria's personal trauma, but an inherited emotional pattern. The therapist helped Maria's Self acknowledge this legacy burden, honoring the strength and resilience of her ancestors while also recognizing that this extreme protection was no longer serving Maria in her current life. By understanding its origin, Maria could, from her Self, gently release this burden, allowing her to ask for support and connect more deeply with others without feeling weak.

Case Example 3: The Burden of "Never Trust Outsiders"

Jamal, a 28-year-old man from a community with a history of systemic discrimination, found it very hard to trust authority figures, even when they seemed helpful. He felt a constant suspicion, a part of him always on guard, whispering, "They will let you down, they are not on your side." He had not experienced direct betrayal from authority figures himself, but his family had many stories of injustice and broken promises from institutions.

Jamal's therapist identified this as a **legacy burden** [22] related to historical trauma and systemic issues. The "Never Trust Outsiders" part was carrying the collective pain and protective wisdom of his community's past experiences. It was a burden absorbed from generations of distrust. The therapist helped Jamal's Self acknowledge this part's protective role, honoring the historical context from which it arose. From this place of understanding, Jamal could, with his Self, begin to differentiate between past collective experiences and his present reality, allowing this part to relax its extreme vigilance and open to the possibility of safe connections in the present, without erasing the important lessons of the past. This approach allowed for a more culturally sensitive healing process.

Key Takeaways

- **All parts have good intentions:** Even extreme or seemingly destructive parts are trying to protect you or manage pain. Approaching them with curiosity and compassion is key to healing.

- **The Self is always present:** Everyone has a core Self that is wise, undamaged, and capable of leading. Learning to tell the difference between true Self-energy and "Self-like parts" is important for both clients and therapists.

- **Burdens can be personal or inherited:** Painful beliefs and emotions can come from your own experiences (personal burdens) or be passed down through family or culture (legacy burdens). Understanding this difference helps guide the healing process.

Chapter 2: Advanced Techniques for Deepening the IFS Process

Moving beyond the first steps of IFS, advanced techniques help you work with the complex and often highly defended inner systems of people who come to therapy with tough problems. These techniques need you to really understand how parts work together and to always be present from your Self.

Working with Dissociated Parts: Reconnecting Fragmented Experiences

When someone goes through trauma, it often leads to dissociation. This is when certain parts of the mind become disconnected from everyday experience, often holding strong emotional burdens and memories. You can think of these dissociated parts like "locked rooms" inside a big house, where the person cannot easily get to them, or it feels too overwhelming to try.

Advanced IFS techniques for working with dissociation involve a careful and gentle way of doing things:

- **Spotting Dissociation:** You learn to notice the small signs that someone is dissociating. This might look like numbness, a person feeling "checked out," or a sudden change in how they feel or act. It is like noticing a faint signal that a part has gone quiet or moved away.

- **Inviting Reconnection:** Instead of trying to force a part to come back, you gently ask the disconnected part to come closer. You might say, "Can you come closer so I can understand you?" This invitation must come from your Self, showing real curiosity and caring. It is like offering a warm hand to a shy animal.

- **Providing Safety:** A calm, caring, and consistently safe therapy space is super important to let these parts know it is okay and safe to step forward and connect. This safety also means going at a slow pace, making sure the person does not get overwhelmed or feel hurt again by suddenly facing intense feelings.

The real challenge in this work is handling the strong emotions that can come up when powerful Exiles start to show themselves, especially in systems that have been carrying heavy burdens for a long time. This means you, as the therapist, need to stay steady and grounded. You can use methods like slow pacing, mindful breathing, and regular safety checks to help keep the person's system stable. For people with Dissociative Identity Disorder (DID), IFS is known as a powerful, evidence-based therapy. The IFS idea of not seeing alters as bad, but as protective parts instead of sick ones, works really well to help them talk to each other and work together more. Your job as the therapist is to help the person's core Self build caring relationships with these alters, which helps them heal and find inner peace.

Let us look at some examples:

Case Example 1: The Frozen Teenager

Sarah, a 28-year-old woman, sought therapy for chronic anxiety and a feeling of being "numb" or "checked out" during stressful situations. She often felt like she was watching her life from a distance. During a session, as she spoke about a difficult childhood memory, her voice became flat, her eyes glazed over, and she seemed to lose touch with her emotions. Her therapist noticed these signs of dissociation.

The therapist, from her Self, gently said, "I notice a part of you seems to have stepped back. Can you tell me, what is that part doing right now? Is it trying to keep you safe?" Sarah, with some effort, said, "It feels like a frozen teenager, hiding in a corner, just trying not to feel anything." The therapist then invited that "frozen teenager" part to come a little closer, assuring it that Sarah's Self and the therapist's Self were there to keep her safe and that she did not have to feel everything all at once. By creating this safe space and inviting the part gently, the frozen part slowly began to show a tiny bit of its fear, a first step toward reconnection.

Case Example 2: The "Floating" Part

Mark, a 40-year-old veteran with a history of combat trauma, often described feeling like he was "floating above his body" when talking about his experiences. This "floating" feeling was a way for a part to escape the intense physical sensations and fear associated with his memories. His therapist recognized this as a dissociative response.

Instead of pushing Mark to "stay in his body," the therapist acknowledged the "floating part" with curiosity. "I notice a part of you goes up and floats when things get intense. What is that part trying to do for you?" The part communicated that it was trying to keep Mark from being overwhelmed, to keep him from feeling the terror in his body. The therapist then asked, "Would that part be willing to just observe from a safe distance, knowing that Mark's Self is here to handle things, and we will go very slowly?" This gentle negotiation, from a place of safety, allowed the "floating part" to relax its extreme role, making it possible for Mark to gradually connect with the sensations in his body without being completely overwhelmed.

Case Example 3: The Silent Child in DID

Maria, a client with Dissociative Identity Disorder (DID), had several alters, but one particular child alter remained completely silent and hidden, even when other alters were present. This "silent child" was believed to hold the most painful, early trauma, and other alters worked hard to keep it hidden. Her therapist understood this as a deeply dissociated part.

The therapist, with Maria's Self, created a very calm and patient environment. They would regularly check in with the silent child, not demanding it speak, but simply offering a consistent, warm presence. "Silent child, we are here. We are not going to push you. We just want you to know you are seen, and we are here when you are ready." Over many sessions, Maria's Self would visualize a safe, cozy space for this child. Eventually, the silent child began to communicate through small gestures, then whispers, and finally, through drawings, slowly revealing its story and allowing for the first steps of healing and communication within Maria's complex internal system.

Unburdening the Exiles: Releasing Deep-Seated Pain

Unburdening is the main healing process in IFS. It is where exiled parts let go of the painful emotions, beliefs, and memories they carry. This leads to real change and personal growth. This process is not just about saying, "Oh, that hurts." It is about actively helping that pain leave.

The advanced way of doing unburdening involves:

- **Building Trust with Protectors:** Before you even get close to an Exile, you must build trust with the Managers and Firefighters who protect it. This makes sure they give you permission and work with you, because they often fear that if the Exile's pain comes out, it will flood the whole system. It is like getting permission from the guards before entering a sensitive area.

- **Witnessing the Pain:** The Exile gets plenty of room and a caring presence to show its hurt, tell its story, and talk about the burdens it has been carrying. The client's Self does this witnessing, and your Self-energy as the therapist supports it. This is not about fixing; it is about truly seeing and hearing.

- **Facilitating Release:** The Self gently guides the Exile to "let go" of its burdens. This can be done with symbolic actions, like imagining the pain melting into light or floating away on a soft breeze. It is a powerful, active step in healing.

- **Integration:** Once a part has let go of its burdens, it can join the inner system in a healthier, more helpful way. It can then use its natural gifts instead of being stuck in a role caused by trauma.

Advanced unburdening methods make sure that no part gets hurt again during this delicate process. For example, someone with PTSD might create a "safe inner room" where an Exile can slowly and safely tell its story, allowing the traumatic material to come out in small, manageable amounts. Your ability as the therapist to pace the work, stay grounded, and do regular safety checks is super important, especially when strong emotions are released during unburdening. The deep healing that happens when burdens are released allows Protectors to relax their extreme watchfulness, leading to a more peaceful and Self-led inner system.

Here are some examples:

Case Example 1: Releasing the Burden of Shame

Michael, a 30-year-old man, carried deep shame about a childhood incident where he was publicly humiliated. This shame was held by an Exile part, and a Manager part worked hard to keep him isolated and avoid social situations to prevent further humiliation. A Firefighter part would sometimes lead him to binge eat when the shame felt too overwhelming.

His therapist first worked with the Manager and Firefighter, acknowledging their protective intent and gaining their permission to approach the shamed Exile. Once the Protectors agreed to step back, Michael's Self approached the Exile. The Exile showed him the memory of the humiliation and the heavy feeling of "I am disgusting" it carried. Michael's Self, with the therapist's support, witnessed this pain fully, offering deep compassion. Then, the Self gently asked the Exile if it was ready to let go of the shame. Michael visualized the shame as a dark, heavy cloak falling off the Exile and dissolving into light. After the unburdening, the Exile felt lighter and more playful, and the Manager and Firefighter parts naturally relaxed their extreme roles, allowing Michael to feel more comfortable in social settings.

Case Example 2: Unburdening the "Unlovable" Exile

Jessica, a 45-year-old woman, struggled with a persistent feeling of being "unlovable," which stemmed from early childhood neglect. This belief was held by an Exile part, and it caused her to push people away (a Manager part) or seek unhealthy relationships (a Firefighter part) to try and prove her worth.

Her therapist helped Jessica's Self connect with the "unlovable" Exile. The Exile showed her images of being alone and longing for connection. Jessica's Self held the Exile with immense compassion, letting it know it was not alone anymore. The Self then asked the Exile if it was ready to release the burden of "unlovable." Jessica, from her Self, imagined gently taking the "unlovable" belief from the Exile and placing it into a beautiful, flowing river, watching it dissolve and be carried away. As the burden left, the Exile felt a sense of peace and lightness. The protective parts, seeing the Exile was no longer carrying such a heavy load, began to trust that Jessica's Self could now attract healthy relationships.

Case Example 3: The PTSD Client's Safe Inner Room

David, a 50-year-old man with complex PTSD from military combat, had an Exile part that held terrifying memories of a specific battle. This Exile was so protected by Firefighters (numbing, avoidance) that any attempt to approach it would lead to intense panic.

His therapist knew that direct, immediate unburdening would be too much. Instead, they focused on creating a "safe inner room" for the Exile. David's Self, with the therapist's guidance, visualized a strong, secure room inside him, with thick walls and a soft, warm light. The therapist then asked the Exile if it would be willing to come into this room, knowing it could leave at any time. Over several sessions, the Exile slowly entered the room. It did not have to tell its whole story at once. Instead, it revealed small pieces, like a single image or a sound, allowing for a titrated (slow and controlled) release of its pain. This careful pacing and consistent safety allowed the Exile to gradually unburden its terror, bit by bit, without overwhelming David's system.

Deepening Self-Leadership: Cultivating Inner Guidance

While basic IFS introduces the idea of the Self, advanced practice focuses on making the Self stronger so it can lead the entire inner system. This is especially important when parts have become too strong because of trauma or ongoing stress. It means helping a person consistently act from their core Self.

Key ways to make Self-leadership stronger include:

- **Consistent Practice of Self-Qualities:** Encourage people to use the 8 Cs (compassion, curiosity, calm, and so on) in their daily lives and when they interact with their parts. Approaching each part with warmth and acceptance, like you would a shy animal, helps build trust inside. This is not just a one-time thing; it is a way of living.

- **Grounded Presence:** When emotions are strong or there is inner conflict, staying grounded through mindful breathing or body scans helps you stay calm. This allows you to make choices from a place of calm awareness, instead of from reactive parts like a frantic Firefighter or a panicky Manager. It is like finding your steady footing in a storm.

- **Differentiating "In Self" from "Self-Led":** A really important difference for advanced therapists is understanding that just being "in Self" (feeling Self qualities for a moment) is different from being "Self-led" (where the Self consistently guides the whole inner system). Being Self-led is the main goal of IFS. It means a big shift towards inner peace and being in charge of your own life.

This strengthening of Self-leadership has big effects on how you handle emotions and how you see yourself, especially in complex PTSD. When the Self takes its rightful place as leader, it can kindly connect with exiled parts, which reduces the extreme actions of protective parts (Managers and Firefighters) and calms emotional distress. This process creates a more organized inner structure, leading to more self-compassion, less self-criticism, and better overall mental well-being. Your ability as the therapist to consistently show and help with Self-leadership helps people become their own healers, so they do not have to rely so much on outside help.

Here are some examples:

Case Example 1: From Overwhelm to Calm Guidance

Sarah, a 30-year-old teacher, often felt overwhelmed by her responsibilities. A "Perfectionist Manager" part pushed her constantly, and when she felt she could not keep up, a "Critic" part would harshly judge her. This led to intense anxiety and feelings of inadequacy. She rarely felt a sense of calm or clarity.

Her therapist helped Sarah practice connecting with her Self by focusing on her breath and noticing the qualities of calm and compassion that were already there. Sarah began to greet her Perfectionist and Critic parts with curiosity, asking, "What are you trying to do for me?" As she consistently practiced this, her Self-energy grew stronger. Instead of being hijacked by anxiety, she could pause, access her Self, and then calmly decide how to approach her tasks, often finding creative solutions her anxious parts could not see. This shift from being driven by parts to being guided by Self was a big step in her emotional regulation.

Case Example 2: Cultivating Courage for Difficult Conversations

Mark, a 45-year-old man, avoided conflict at all costs. A "People-Pleaser Manager" part kept him from speaking his truth, fearing rejection. This led to resentment and a feeling of being unheard. He wanted to set boundaries but felt paralyzed by fear.

His therapist helped Mark identify the "People-Pleaser" part and the fear it carried. They also focused on cultivating the Self-quality of **Courage**. Mark practiced small acts of courage in his daily life, like expressing a mild preference. His therapist helped him see that true courage was not about being fearless, but about acting from Self even when a part felt scared. As Mark's Self-leadership deepened, he could approach his "People-Pleaser" part with compassion, letting it know that his Self could handle any discomfort that came from setting boundaries. This allowed him to have a difficult but necessary conversation with a family member, feeling grounded and clear, rather than anxious and resentful.

Case Example 3: Self-Led Parenting

Maria, a new mother, found herself reacting impulsively to her toddler's tantrums, often yelling or withdrawing, and then feeling immense guilt. She felt controlled by a "Frustrated Firefighter" part and a "Guilty Exile." She longed to be a calm, patient parent but felt unable to.

Her therapist helped Maria understand that her reactions came from parts trying to cope with overwhelm and unhealed Exiles from her own childhood. The therapist guided Maria to practice Self-leadership by pausing before reacting to her child's cries. Maria would place a hand on her heart, take a few slow breaths, and ask, "What part of me is activated right now? What does my Self want to do?" This simple practice, done consistently, allowed her Self to come forward. From her Self, Maria could then approach her frustrated parts with compassion, and then respond to her child from a place of calm and connection, rather than reactivity. This deepened her self-compassion and improved her relationship with her child, showing the power of Self-leadership in real-time parenting.

Mapping the System: Charting the Internal Landscape

While basic IFS might just involve naming a few important parts, advanced practice uses a full system map to chart the entire inner world. This includes all the complex relationships between parts and the specific burdens they carry. This process gives you a clear picture, both visually and in your mind, which is super helpful when working with complex cases.

How to make a system map:

- **Detailed Part Identification:** List all the Managers, Firefighters, and Exiles you have found. Write down their traits, what they believe, and what they do. It is like making a roster of all the players on a team.

- **Identifying Connections and Relationships:** Draw lines or arrows to show how different protectors defend specific exiles, how parts are against each other (polarized), and how they interact within the system. For example, a Manager that always wants things perfect might protect an Exile that feels "unlovable." Then, a Firefighter might use late-night snacks to numb the pain when that "unlovable" Exile gets activated.

- **Visual Representation:** Use drawings, flowcharts, or even computer tools (like the IFS Guide App) to make a picture of the inner system. This turns a "mental mess into an organized structure," helping both you and your client understand the inner workings much better.

The real value of mapping the system is that it shows you complex connections and old patterns that might otherwise stay hidden. This clear picture helps you, the therapist, plan more exact and effective ways to help. You can target the real causes of distress instead of just dealing with the surface problems. It helps you find the key spots within the system where you can make the biggest difference in healing.

Here are some examples:

Case Example 1: Mapping the Anxiety Cycle

David, a 25-year-old student, suffered from severe social anxiety. He would avoid social gatherings (a Manager part), and when forced into them, he would experience panic attacks (a Firefighter part). He felt a deep sense of inadequacy (an Exile part).

His therapist guided David in mapping his system. They drew a diagram:

- **Exile:** A small, scared child part, burdened with "I am not good enough," from early school experiences.
- **Manager:** A "Social Avoider" part, which kept David home, believing it was protecting the child from judgment.
- **Firefighter:** A "Panic Attack" part, which would flood David with physical symptoms (racing heart, shortness of breath) when the Social Avoider failed, trying to make him escape the situation quickly. The map clearly showed how the Social Avoider tried to prevent the Exile's pain, and how the Panic Attack Firefighter would take over when the Manager's strategy failed. This visual clarity helped David see the cycle and understand that his parts were trying to help, even if their methods were distressing.

Case Example 2: Charting the Self-Sabotage System

Maria, a 35-year-old professional, repeatedly sabotaged her career success. She would get close to promotions, then suddenly make mistakes or withdraw. She felt a deep sense of unworthiness and a fear of success.

Through system mapping, Maria and her therapist charted:

- **Exile:** A young part, burdened with "I don't deserve good things," from a childhood where success was met with jealousy or punishment.

- **Manager:** A "Self-Saboteur" part, which would create mistakes or withdrawal, believing it was protecting the Exile from the dangers of success.
- **Firefighter:** A "Numbing" part, which would lead to excessive TV watching or oversleeping after a self-sabotaging act, trying to dull the pain of perceived failure or the fear of success. The map showed how the Self-Saboteur was actually a protector, and how the Numbing Firefighter would step in. This clear picture helped Maria see the hidden logic of her self-sabotage, allowing her to approach these parts with curiosity and begin to change the pattern.

Case Example 3: Visualizing the Chronic Pain System

John, a 50-year-old man, experienced chronic back pain that doctors could not fully explain. He also had a strong "Stoic Manager" part that told him to "just push through" the pain, and a "Frustrated Firefighter" part that would lead to angry outbursts when the pain became unbearable.

His therapist helped John map his internal system in relation to his pain:

- **Exile:** A young, vulnerable part that held the burden of "I am broken" and deep sadness about his physical limitations. This part also held the physical sensation of pain.
- **Manager:** The "Stoic" part, which tried to control the pain by ignoring it and pushing John to keep working, believing it was protecting him from feeling weak or useless.

- **Firefighter:** The "Angry Outburst" part, which would explode when the Stoic Manager could no longer contain the pain, trying to release the overwhelming frustration and helplessness. The map showed how the Stoic Manager's efforts to suppress the pain actually made the Frustrated Firefighter more likely to erupt. By seeing this visual, John understood that his pain was not just physical; it was connected to his inner parts and their protective strategies. This new understanding opened the door to working with the parts directly, rather than just trying to manage the pain itself.

Working with Polarized Parts: Resolving Internal Conflicts

Polarization happens when two or more parts inside a person have opposite goals or ways of doing things. This creates inner conflict that can feel impossible to solve. These conflicts often come from trauma, where different parts take on extreme roles to try and protect the system.

Advanced ways to work with polarized parts include:

- **Allowing Each Side to Speak:** Create a safe space where both polarized parts can express their worries, fears, and what they think, without being interrupted or judged. This makes sure that each part feels heard and understood. It is like giving each side of an argument a chance to present its case fully.

- **Mediation by Self:** The client's Self, guided by your Self-energy as the therapist, helps the parts talk to each other. This builds mutual understanding and caring between them. The Self's presence helps calm the conflict and creates a chance for them to find a solution. The Self acts as a wise, neutral mediator.

- **Facilitating Compromise and Collaboration:** Guide the parts towards a middle ground or a new way of working together that respects the good intentions of both. This might mean one part softens its demands while the other takes small, brave steps forward. It is about finding a win-win solution where all parts feel respected.

This way of working is especially helpful in couples therapy, where partners often show their inner polarizations outside, leading to arguments. For example, one partner's inner Firefighter might clash with the other partner's inner Protector, which then makes each other's Exiles feel hurt again. By finding these patterns, IFS helps partners talk from their Self, saying things like, "A part of me feels really hurt when you're silent," instead of angrily saying, "You always ignore me!" This moves the focus from blaming to understanding inner workings, which helps build healthier relationships both inside and with others.

Here are some examples:

Case Example 1: The "Achiever" vs. "Relaxer" Polarization

Sarah, a successful lawyer, felt constantly torn between a part that pushed her to achieve more (an "Achiever Manager") and a part that craved rest and relaxation (a "Relaxer Firefighter"). This led to burnout, guilt when she rested, and frustration when she was not productive. These two parts were deeply polarized.

Her therapist helped Sarah's Self invite both parts to speak. The "Achiever" expressed its fear of failure and poverty, believing that constant work was the only way to be safe. The "Relaxer" expressed its exhaustion and fear of collapsing if it did not get rest. Sarah's Self listened with compassion to both. Then, the Self mediated, helping the parts see their shared goal: Sarah's well-being. They found a compromise: the "Achiever" agreed to schedule specific, protected rest times, and the "Relaxer" agreed to be more present and less demanding during work hours. This collaboration allowed Sarah to be both productive and rested, reducing her inner conflict.

Case Example 2: The "Confronter" vs. "Avoider" Polarization

Mark struggled in his relationships because a "Confronter Firefighter" part would lash out aggressively when he felt hurt, while an "Avoider Manager" part would then shut down completely, leading to unresolved conflicts. He felt stuck in a cycle of anger and withdrawal.

His therapist helped Mark's Self bring the "Confronter" and "Avoider" parts into dialogue. The "Confronter" explained it was trying to protect Mark from being taken advantage of, believing aggression was the only way to be heard. The "Avoider" explained it was trying to prevent further pain and conflict, believing withdrawal was the safest option. Mark's Self helped them understand each other's positive intentions. The Self then guided them to a new strategy: the "Confronter" agreed to express hurt calmly from Self, and the "Avoider" agreed to stay present and listen, knowing Mark's Self could handle the discomfort. This allowed Mark to communicate his needs effectively without resorting to extreme reactions.

Case Example 3: Couples Therapy: The "Critic" and the "Sensitive One"

In couples therapy, Lisa often criticized her husband, Tom, for being "lazy" (a "Critic Manager" part). Tom, in response, would withdraw and become sullen (a "Sensitive Exile" protected by a "Withdrawer Firefighter"). This created a painful cycle in their marriage.

Their therapist helped Lisa identify her "Critic" part and Tom his "Withdrawer" and "Sensitive" parts. The therapist explained that Lisa's Critic was trying to motivate Tom (positive intent), but its method was hurting Tom's Sensitive Exile. Tom's Withdrawer was trying to protect his Sensitive Exile from further pain. From their respective Selves, Lisa learned to say, "A part of me feels worried about our finances and wants to see more action," instead of "You're so lazy!" Tom, from his Self, could then hear Lisa's concern without his Sensitive Exile being triggered as intensely, and his Withdrawer part could relax. This shift from parts-driven blame to Self-led communication transformed their arguments into opportunities for understanding and collaboration.

Key Takeaways

- **Dissociation is a protector's strategy:** When parts disconnect, they are trying to keep you safe from overwhelming pain. Approach them gently, inviting them to reconnect from a place of safety and curiosity.
- **Unburdening is active release:** It is not just about talking about pain, but actively helping exiled parts let

go of their heavy emotional loads. Building trust with protectors first is essential for this deep healing.

- **Self-leadership is a daily practice:** Consistently using your Self-qualities and staying grounded helps your Self guide your inner system, leading to better emotional regulation and a stronger sense of who you are.

- **Mapping brings clarity:** Drawing out your inner parts and their connections helps you see complex patterns and plan more effective ways to help your system work together.

- **Polarization can be resolved:** Inner conflicts between parts can be healed by letting each part speak, mediating with your Self, and finding new ways for them to work together towards a shared positive goal.

Chapter 3: IFS in Complex Trauma and Dissociative Disorders

When we talk about healing deep wounds, especially those from long-term, repeated harms, we are often talking about **complex trauma (CPTSD)**. This kind of trauma usually happens when a person is young, leading to a fragmented inner system and big struggles with managing feelings and relating to others [4, 57, 58, 59]. IFS offers a powerful and effective way to help with CPTSD. It is different from other ways of working because it welcomes even the most extreme symptoms right from the start, seeing them as helpers, not as something wrong [4].

Complex Trauma (CPTSD): A Systemic Approach to Deep Healing

IFS helps with CPTSD by taking a special approach:

- **Not labeling symptoms as bad:** Think of extreme symptoms—like self-harm, thoughts of ending it all, or addictions—not as signs of something wrong with the person, but as desperate attempts by protective parts to handle overwhelming pain and shield vulnerable Exiles [4, 7, 8]. This kind and understanding view helps people feel safe enough to open up and begin healing.

- **Connecting directly with Protectors:** Instead of waiting to build up lots of coping skills before dealing with hard memories, IFS welcomes those extreme symptoms and tries to learn about their good intentions [4, 8]. This means asking for their permission to get close to the painful wounds. This builds trust inside and makes protective parts less resistant [4].

- **Helping the nervous system calm down:** IFS helps people notice and work with fears tied to traumatic memories and strong feelings [4, 25]. This allows them to use calming skills and go at a slow pace so they do not get overwhelmed. This is super important for people whose nervous systems are always on high alert or react too strongly because of long-term trauma [4, 25].

- **Witnessing and Unburdening:** IFS creates a space where people can truly witness their own stories with Self-compassion [4, 21]. This leads to the **unburdening process,** where painful beliefs and memories are finally released [4, 21]. This hands-on process helps them reprocess those memories and grow in self-compassion, freeing parts from their extreme, trauma-based roles [4].

- **Bringing back Self-Leadership:** By making the Self's presence stronger, IFS helps to bring harmony to the inner system [4, 25]. This reduces the extreme actions of protective parts and allows for kind connection with exiled parts that carry the weight of trauma [4, 25]. This directly addresses problems with managing feelings and negative self-talk, which are big parts of CPTSD [4, 57].

Let us look at some examples:

Case Example 1: Softening the Self-Harm Protector

Sarah, a 28-year-old, came to therapy with a history of self-harm, a behavior she used when feeling overwhelmed by intense emotional pain. She felt immense shame about it and believed it was a sign of her weakness.

Her therapist, using an IFS approach, did not try to stop the self-harm directly. Instead, she asked Sarah, "Is there a part of you that makes you do this?" Sarah identified a "Cutter" part. The therapist, from her Self, asked, "What is the Cutter trying to do for you?" The Cutter, surprisingly, showed that it was trying to release overwhelming emotional pressure, a desperate Firefighter [7, 8]. It feared that if the pressure built up too much, Sarah would explode or vanish. The therapist acknowledged this protective intent: "I see you're trying to save Sarah from feeling too much. That's a powerful job." By welcoming the Cutter and understanding its positive intent, Sarah's Self could then negotiate with it, promising to find other ways to manage the pressure, like connecting with a "Breathe" part or a "Grounding" part. This built trust, allowing the Cutter to gradually relax its extreme vigilance, and paving the way for Sarah's Self to approach the Exile holding the overwhelming pain.

Case Example 2: From Hyper-Vigilance to Inner Calm

Mark, a 45-year-old, lived with constant hyper-vigilance and anxiety, a result of prolonged childhood abuse. He was always on edge, scanning for danger, and easily startled. His nervous system felt perpetually stuck in "fight or flight."

His therapist recognized that Mark's hyper-vigilance was controlled by a Manager part, trying to predict and prevent future harm, protecting a terrified Exile [4, 25]. Instead of trying to force Mark to relax, the therapist worked with the Manager, acknowledging its tireless efforts. "You've worked so hard to keep Mark safe, always on watch. That must be exhausting." This validation helped the Manager feel seen.

The therapist then helped Mark's Self explore what the Manager feared most. It feared being caught off guard, a feeling connected to old trauma memories. The therapist helped Mark's Self invite calming strategies, like mindful breathing, into the system, reassuring the Manager that the Self could handle the sensations [4, 25]. Slowly, the Manager began to trust the Self's ability to regulate the nervous system, allowing Mark to experience moments of calm and safety he had not felt in years.

Case Example 3: Healing the "Unlovable" Burden in CPTSD

Maria, a 35-year-old, struggled with a deep-seated belief that she was "unlovable," stemming from years of emotional neglect and criticism. This belief was held by a core Exile, which was heavily protected by a "Self-Critic" Manager and a "Withdrawal" Firefighter.

Her therapist helped Maria's Self approach the Self-Critic, understanding its intent to "fix" Maria so she would be loved. Then, the therapist gained permission from the Manager to connect with the Exile. Maria's Self, with the therapist's steady presence, gently welcomed the "Unlovable" Exile [4, 21]. The Exile revealed painful memories of being ignored and told she was "too much." Maria's Self compassionately witnessed these memories, feeling the Exile's profound loneliness and sadness. Then, Maria's Self offered to unburden the "unlovable" belief. Maria visualized the belief as a heavy, gray cloud surrounding the Exile, which slowly dissolved as her Self wrapped the Exile in warmth and love. The Exile, now unburdened, transformed into a part that felt inherently worthy of connection. This profound shift changed Maria's relationship with herself and others, reducing her negative self-concept and improving her affect regulation [4, 57].

Dissociative Disorders (DID): Fostering Internal Harmony and Integration

Dissociative Identity Disorder (DID) is a condition where a person has two or more distinct identities, or "alters," inside them [20, 26, 27, 28]. These alters often show up as a way to cope with very severe and long-term childhood trauma [20, 23]. IFS is known as a strong, evidence-based therapy for dissociative disorders [23].

IFS has a special way of handling the complexities of DID:

- **Not seeing alters as bad:** IFS sees alters not as something wrong or sick, but as separate sub-personalities or "parts" that have taken on extreme protective roles to handle overwhelming trauma [23, 24, 28]. This non-judgmental stance is super important for building trust with these parts, which are often very cautious and guarded [23].

- **Helping alters talk to each other:** Therapy focuses on understanding and healing these inner parts by helping the person's core Self build a kind and understanding relationship with all their different identities [23]. The Self acts as the main, unifying presence that can talk to and mediate between the different identities [23].

- **Helping inner harmony and integration:** The main goal is to help the person connect with their core Self and use its natural qualities (calm, curiosity, compassion) to heal and put together the parts that carry the burden of trauma [23, 24]. This process helps them work better together and feel more like a whole person, so they do not need to rely on dissociation as a way to cope [23].

- **Creating Safety:** Because the exiled parts in DID are often very vulnerable, making sure the therapy space is consistently safe is super important [20, 23]. This allows dissociative parts to slowly share their stories without feeling overwhelmed or re-traumatized [23, 25]. Your Self-led presence and careful pacing are vital in this process [25].

Let us look at some examples:

Case Example 1: Introducing the Core Self to a System

David, a 40-year-old with DID, presented with several distinct alters, including a fierce "Gatekeeper" who controlled access to other parts and a frightened "Child" part that rarely spoke. His system was highly guarded, making it hard to make progress.

His therapist began by first acknowledging the Gatekeeper's protective role, without trying to bypass it. "I see how hard you work to keep David safe, making sure no one gets hurt. I respect that." The therapist, from their own calm Self, then introduced the concept of David's own core Self to the Gatekeeper. "David has a calm, wise Self inside, just like you have been protecting. Would you be willing to allow David's Self to be present here with us, to help you in your job?" The Gatekeeper, feeling respected and not challenged, slowly allowed David's Self to be more present. From this Self-led place, David could then begin to relate to his other alters, not as fragmented identities, but as parts of himself, starting with compassionate curiosity towards the frightened Child part [23].

Case Example 2: Mediating Internal Conflicts Between Alters

Lisa, a 30-year-old with DID, experienced frequent internal arguments between a "Responsible Adult" alter who focused on daily tasks and a "Rebellious Teenager" alter who would often sabotage her efforts, leading to missed appointments and outbursts. This inner conflict caused significant distress.

Her therapist helped Lisa recognize that these were both parts trying to help her, but with opposing strategies [23]. The Responsible Adult wanted stability, fearing chaos. The Rebellious Teenager felt stifled and unheard, trying to gain freedom. The therapist, from her Self, helped Lisa's core Self mediate between these two alters. "Responsible Adult, what do you fear if Lisa gives the Teenager some space? Rebellious Teenager, what do you truly need that you're not getting?" By allowing each alter to voice its perspective, and by providing a Self-led presence that honored both, Lisa's Self could help them find common ground. They eventually agreed that the Responsible Adult would schedule some "fun time" for the Teenager each week, and in return, the Teenager would cooperate with daily responsibilities, leading to a significant reduction in internal conflict and external sabotage [23].

Case Example 3: Gradual Unburdening of a Traumatized Child Alter

Mark, a 50-year-old with DID, had a "Small Child" alter that held severe trauma from early abuse. This alter would cause flashbacks and intense emotional distress whenever it was close to the surface, leading a powerful "Protector" alter to keep it hidden at all costs.

His therapist understood the Protector's intention to prevent Mark from experiencing overwhelming pain. The therapist first built a strong alliance with the Protector, acknowledging its fierce loyalty and the heavy burden it carried. "You've done an incredible job protecting Mark from this pain for so long." With the Protector's permission, and in a carefully paced manner, the therapist helped Mark's Self create an "inner safe place" for the Small Child [25]. Mark's Self, with constant reassurance from the therapist, gradually approached the Small Child. The Small Child, feeling the consistent safety and compassion from Mark's Self, slowly began to show fragmented memories of the abuse. Mark's Self, with the therapist's co-regulation, witnessed the Small Child's pain, validating its experience without becoming overwhelmed [23]. This gentle witnessing led to the gradual unburdening of the trauma, allowing the Small Child to feel safe enough to release its burdens, and the Protector to relax its extreme role, fostering greater integration within Mark's system [23].

A Thought on Resilience

Working with complex trauma and dissociative disorders requires patience, compassion, and a steady hand. It is a journey of uncovering hidden strengths and helping people reconnect with their own amazing capacity for healing. This work reminds us that even after the deepest hurts, the Self remains whole, ready to guide the way to inner harmony.

Key Takeaways

- **CPTSD: Symptoms are Protectors:** In CPTSD, extreme symptoms are attempts by parts to cope with overwhelming pain. Welcome these parts, understand their intent, and work with them from your Self.

- **CPTSD: Self-Leadership Heals:** Strengthening the Self helps regulate the nervous system, witness trauma, unburden pain, and improve self-concept.

- **DID: Alters are Protectors:** View alters not as pathology, but as parts that protected against severe trauma. This non-judgmental stance builds trust.

- **DID: Self Unifies:** The core Self fosters communication and mediates between alters, promoting harmony and gradual integration of identity.

- **DID: Safety First:** A consistently safe therapeutic environment and careful pacing are essential for parts to reveal and heal their traumatic stories without re-traumatization.

Chapter 4: IFS in Addiction Treatment

Healing the Roots of Compulsion

Thinking about addiction often brings up ideas of moral failings or a lack of willpower. But Internal Family Systems therapy offers a different, much more understanding way to look at it [6, 31, 60, 72, 73]. IFS sees addictive behaviors not as something wrong with the person, but as attempts by "protective parts" to handle emotional pain or inner struggles [6, 74]. This view, rooted in understanding trauma, shifts our focus from just trying to stop the addictive behavior to healing the deeper wounds that are actually driving those powerful urges [6].

Understanding Addictive Behaviors as Protection

IFS starts with a powerful idea: **addictive behaviors are really just protection**. These behaviors, often driven by **"Firefighter" parts** that jump in impulsively when things feel bad, or **"Manager" parts** trying to control inner states, are strategies developed by parts to shield the person from deeper emotional pain, past trauma, or to silence a harsh inner critic [6, 31, 60, 74]. This way of looking at things truly shows that there are **"no bad parts,"** even the ones doing seemingly harmful things [6, 7, 8]. Every part, even an addictive one, is trying its best to help, often in a misguided way.

Identifying and Differentiating Addictive Parts

A key step in using IFS for addiction is helping people identify these protective parts and understand the good intentions behind what they are doing [6, 74]. This allows people to **"unblend" from them.** Think of it like stepping back from a painting to see the whole picture instead of being right up close to one brushstroke. You can observe these behaviors without feeling completely taken over by them or believing that is all you are [6]. This step creates the space needed for real healing to begin.

Fostering Self-Leadership

A central aim in this work is to help people connect with their true **Self** [6]. The Self is naturally compassionate, curious, and calm. From this Self-led place, people can approach their addictive parts and the wounded parts underneath with understanding and kindness, rather than judgment [6]. It is like having a wise, loving parent inside who can finally talk to the struggling children.

Healing Underlying Wounds (Unburdening)

Addiction almost always comes from unresolved trauma and emotional pain carried by "wounded parts" or Exiles [6, 74]. IFS really focuses on giving these hurting parts the space to heal and be heard through the **unburdening process** [6, 74]. This means releasing the emotional pain and extreme beliefs that are feeding the addiction. It is like finally emptying those heavy backpacks of pain that the parts have been carrying for so long.

Promoting Self-Regulation and Internal Harmony

As wounded parts heal and protective parts change their extreme roles, people start to develop healthier ways to cope and feel a deeper sense of well-being [6]. This leads to a more harmonious inner system, where there is trust in the person's ability to lead their own life without needing outside substances or behaviors to numb their feelings [6]. This approach truly helps people take back control and make choices that match who they really are, their authentic Self.

Let us look at some examples:

Case Example 1: The "Numbing" Firefighter

Michael, a 38-year-old, struggled with alcohol addiction. He would drink heavily whenever he felt stressed, anxious, or lonely. He hated his drinking and felt like a failure.

His therapist, using IFS, helped Michael see his drinking not as a moral failing, but as a behavior driven by a "Numbing" Firefighter part [6, 74]. This part was reacting impulsively to overwhelm, trying to extinguish intense feelings of anxiety and loneliness that were held by an Exile. Michael's Self approached the Numbing part with curiosity: "What are you trying to do for me when I drink?" The Numbing part revealed its fear that if Michael felt the loneliness, he would be crushed. By understanding this protective intent, Michael's Self could thank the Numbing part for its effort and gently ask it to step back. This allowed Michael's Self to approach the Lonely Exile, witness its pain, and unburden the feeling of being utterly alone. As the Exile healed, the Numbing part's urge to drink lessened, and Michael found healthier ways to cope with stress.

Case Example 2: The "Control" Manager and the "Chaos" Exile

Sarah, a 30-year-old, had an eating disorder, restricting her food intake to feel a sense of control. This behavior was driven by a "Control" Manager part, which believed it was keeping her safe from inner "Chaos," an Exile part holding feelings of helplessness from childhood trauma.

Her therapist helped Sarah's Self connect with the Control Manager, acknowledging its positive intent to maintain order. "You work so hard to keep Sarah safe and in control. What are you afraid would happen if you relaxed?" The Manager revealed its terror of the "Chaos" Exile overwhelming Sarah. Sarah's Self then engaged with the Chaos Exile, which held profound feelings of powerlessness from a chaotic upbringing. Through witnessing and unburdening, the Chaos Exile released its burden, feeling seen and cared for by Sarah's Self. As the Exile healed, the Control Manager softened its rigid grip, allowing Sarah to relax her eating rules and find a more balanced approach to food, no longer needing to micromanage her inner state.

Case Example 3: The "Punisher" and the "Rebellion"

David, a 45-year-old, was addicted to gambling. He often felt a powerful urge to gamble when he was feeling low or criticized himself harshly. He had an inner "Punisher" part that constantly told him he was worthless, and a "Rebellion" Firefighter part that would then seek out risky, self-destructive behaviors like gambling to defy the Punisher.

His therapist helped David's Self identify the Punisher as a Manager part, trying to motivate him by criticism, and the Rebellion as a Firefighter, reacting to the pain caused by the Punisher, protecting an Exile that felt inherently bad [6, 74]. David's Self first dialogued with the Punisher, understanding its fear that David would never be good enough without its harsh critiques. Then, the Self connected with the Rebellion, seeing its desperate attempt to feel powerful against the inner torment. Finally, David's Self approached the "Bad" Exile, witnessing the deep shame it carried. By unburdening this shame, and by the Self offering compassion to the

Punisher and the Rebellion, the parts began to transform. The Punisher softened its voice, and the Rebellion found healthier ways to express independence, leading to a significant reduction in the urge to gamble.

A Look Ahead

IFS offers a way to move beyond just managing symptoms in addiction. It helps people heal the very roots of their suffering, allowing their true Self to emerge and guide them towards lasting well-being. This deeper healing frees them to build a life no longer driven by compulsion.

Chapter 5: IFS Integration with Other Advanced Modalities

The beauty of IFS is how well it blends with other helpful therapy approaches [29]. When you combine IFS with other proven methods, especially for those with really complex problems, you get a powerful set of tools. It is like having different specialists on a team, all working together for the best outcome.

EMDR (Eye Movement Desensitization and Reprocessing)

Putting IFS together with **EMDR** creates a very strong way to heal complex trauma [5, 33]. EMDR helps process traumatic memories by using eye movements or other back-and-forth stimulation [5]. IFS makes EMDR even better by:

- **Making things safe and steady:** IFS gives you a gentle way to understand and work with protective parts *before* you even start the deeper trauma work with EMDR [5]. This helps people build trust inside themselves and feel safe, making the EMDR process easier to handle and less overwhelming, especially for those with very strong protective parts [5].

- **Finding the parts that hold trauma:** IFS helps people figure out which specific parts are holding those trauma-related memories [5]. This means EMDR can be more focused and effective.

- **Reducing resistance:** Sometimes, parts might resist EMDR because they are afraid of overwhelming pain [5]. IFS lets you talk to these parts, reassure them, and get their permission before you start EMDR [5].

This approach respects the person's inner system and ensures everyone is "on board."

- **Better processing:** During EMDR, people might come across strong feelings, memories, or beliefs held by different parts [5]. Using IFS ideas during EMDR sessions means you can connect with these parts kindly and without judgment. This helps in deeper healing and brings new, helpful information from the Self to those parts [5].

Let us look at some examples:

Case Example 1: Preparing a Fearful Protector for EMDR

Sarah had a history of severe childhood neglect, and an "Avoidance" Manager part would shut her down whenever the topic of her past came up. Her therapist felt EMDR could help process the trauma, but the Avoidance part was a big obstacle.

The therapist used IFS to first talk to the Avoidance Manager. "I see you're trying to protect Sarah from the pain of those memories. What are you afraid will happen if she looks at them?" The Avoidance part showed a fear of Sarah being completely overwhelmed and falling apart. Sarah's Self, with the therapist's guidance, then reassured the Avoidance part: "My Self is here, and I will keep us grounded. We will go slowly, and if it gets too much, we will stop." With the Avoidance part's hesitant permission, and a clear signal system for stopping, EMDR processing could begin. The Avoidance part, feeling respected and heard, was able to relax enough for Sarah to start processing the traumatic memories safely.

Case Example 2: Working with Emerging Exiles During EMDR

During an EMDR session, Mark was processing a specific combat memory. Suddenly, he became very tearful and a new, childlike voice emerged, saying, "I'm so scared! Where's my mom?" This was a young Exile coming forward.

Instead of continuing the EMDR without interruption, the therapist paused the bilateral stimulation and, from their Self, gently turned to the emerging Exile, using IFS principles. "Little one, I see you're here. What do you need right now?" Mark's Self, with the therapist's support, was able to offer comfort and compassion to this scared child part, letting it know it was safe in the present. Once the Exile felt seen and soothed by the Self, the therapist could then ask if it was okay to resume EMDR to process the broader memory, now with the Self holding the Exile. This integration allowed for a much deeper and more complete processing of the trauma.

Case Example 3: Addressing Resistance to EMDR Desensitization

Lisa had a "Skeptical" part that resisted the EMDR process, particularly the idea of her brain processing trauma. It kept saying, "This won't work. It's just silly." This resistance was stalling her progress.

Her therapist used IFS to directly address the Skeptical part. "Skeptical part, I hear your doubts. What are you worried about if this EMDR does work, or if it doesn't?" The Skeptical part revealed a fear of false hope, having been disappointed by other therapies before, and a deeper fear of truly healing, which would mean letting go of its protective, familiar role. Lisa's Self acknowledged these fears. The therapist then asked the Skeptical part if it would be willing to just observe, staying in the background, rather than actively sabotaging, for a short period. By honoring its concerns and negotiating with it, the Skeptical part agreed to allow the EMDR process to continue, albeit with an watchful eye. This consent-based approach reduced the internal struggle and allowed Lisa to engage more fully with the EMDR.

Somatic Experiencing (SE) and Polyvagal Theory

Putting IFS together with ways that focus on the body, like **Somatic Experiencing (SE)** and **Polyvagal Theory**, often called **Somatic IFS**, means we understand that trauma does not just live in the mind—it lives in the body too [29, 34, 35, 36, 37]. This combined approach gives us a deeper way to heal complex trauma by looking at how distress shows up in the body [29].

Here are the key strategies and benefits of this combination:

- **More Body Awareness:** Somatic IFS helps people become more aware of what is happening in their bodies [29]. They can start to notice how Manager parts might make their body tense, how Firefighter parts cause numbness, and how Exiles hold onto frozen body stories from trauma [29].

- **Calming the Nervous System:** Simple practices like mindful breathing and other body-focused exercises can activate the vagus nerve, which helps the body calm down [36, 37]. This reduces stress hormones and helps the body's natural regulation system get back on track [36, 37]. It helps people move out of "fight/flight" states (too active) or "freeze/numb" states (too shut down) [36, 37].

- **Embodied Self-Energy:** This approach stresses that the Self's calming energy needs to be felt in the body to be truly powerful [29, 35]. This allows the Self to connect with and support those parts that are either too worked up or too shut down [29, 35].

- **Processing Hidden Memories:** By focusing on body signals and movements, people can process traumatic memories that are stored in ways they do not consciously remember [29]. This allows the body to release stored trauma, which can be called **physiological unburdening** [29]. This makes therapy feel less threatening and more effective, especially for people with very hard mental health problems.

- **Supportive Touch and Movement:** Practices like caring touch (imagined or real, always led by the client) and expressive movement can give people new, healing experiences [29]. This can release oxytocin, a calming hormone, and help regulate the nervous system, undoing the physical effects of trauma [29].

Let us look at some examples:

Case Example 1: Releasing Body Tension from an Overwhelmed Manager

Anna, a 40-year-old, suffered from chronic neck and shoulder pain, which worsened with stress. She had a "Pushing" Manager part that kept her working long hours, and her body often felt stiff and rigid.

Her therapist, using Somatic IFS, first helped Anna's Self connect with the Pushing Manager. It revealed it was terrified of Anna failing or being seen as weak, leading to constant tension. Instead of just talking, the therapist guided Anna to notice the specific sensations in her neck and shoulders. Anna's Self then gently placed a hand on her neck and, from a place of compassion, asked the tense Manager part, "What if you could let just 5% of this tension go? What might happen then?" As Anna's Self offered this gentle invitation, her Pushing Manager, feeling seen and supported, allowed a subtle softening in her muscles. This bodily release, driven by Self-energy, was a **physiological unburdening**, showing the Manager that relaxing did not mean failure [29].

Case Example 2: Befriending a Frozen Exile in the Body

John, a 30-year-old, felt numb and disconnected from his body, particularly in his legs, after a traumatic accident. He had an Exile part that seemed "frozen" in the memory of the impact, leading to a sense of unreality.

His therapist, using Somatic IFS, helped John's Self gently bring awareness to his legs, not to force sensation, but just to "be with" the numbness. John's Self asked the frozen Exile, "What are you holding onto in my legs?" The Exile showed him a flash of the accident, and a deep sense of helplessness. The therapist then guided John's Self to slowly, almost imperceptibly, make tiny, gentle movements with his toes, inviting "pendulation"—a subtle movement between sensation and calm [34, 35]. As the Self stayed present and embodied, the frozen Exile gradually released tiny tremors and warmth in his legs. This somatic processing allowed the Exile to move out of its frozen state, releasing the implicit memory of helplessness and bringing more feeling and connection back to John's body [29].

Case Example 3: Calming Hyper-Arousal with Polyvagal-Informed IFS

Maria, a 25-year-old, experienced frequent panic attacks and felt her heart race constantly, a symptom of her hyper-vigilant nervous system due to complex trauma. Her "Fear" Firefighter part was always on high alert.

Her therapist used Polyvagal-informed IFS to help Maria's Self activate her ventral vagal pathway [36, 37]. First, they noticed the "Fear" Firefighter and understood its positive intent to warn Maria of danger. Then, the therapist guided Maria's Self to engage in slow, deliberate exhalations, humming, and gentle eye movements, practices that directly stimulate the vagus nerve [36, 37]. As Maria's nervous system began to calm, her Self approached the Fear Firefighter. "It's okay now. My Self is here, and my body is feeling safer. You can rest." This active, embodied Self-presence helped the Fear Firefighter relax its extreme role, allowing Maria's nervous system to shift out of hyper-arousal and into a calmer, more regulated state, significantly reducing the frequency and intensity of her panic attacks [29, 36, 37].

Dialectical Behavior Therapy (DBT)

DBT gives people really practical skills for managing emotional storms and getting better at dealing with others [38, 39]. But sometimes, people find it hard to use these skills all the time if there are deeper emotional wounds that have not healed [38]. This is where IFS comes in, helping DBT by:

- **Healing Core Emotional Hurts:** While DBT offers solid skills for handling distress and strong emotions, IFS goes deeper [38, 39]. It works on healing the parts that are carrying the underlying pain that makes it tough to use those skills. This means moving beyond just coping to getting truly, lasting healing [38].

- **Using skills with parts in mind:** Instead of simply trying to distract from overwhelming emotions, IFS encourages you to ask, "Which part is overwhelmed, and what does it need?" [38, 39] This allows for a kind and understanding response to the part that is hurting, making DBT skills feel more natural and easier to stick with.

- **Changing self-criticism:** DBT encourages you to challenge those harsh self-critical thoughts [38]. IFS takes this a step further by inviting you to talk to the critical part itself, understand its fears, and offer it compassion so it can soften its harshness [38].

- **Handling resistance to skills:** If a part does not want to use DBT skills, IFS provides a way to talk to that part, reassure it, and get its agreement [38, 39]. This makes sure that the person's inner system is on board with the therapy goals.

Let us look at some examples:

Case Example 1: Understanding Why a Part Resists Distress Tolerance Skills

Sarah, a client struggling with intense emotional dysregulation, was taught DBT's distress tolerance skills but found herself unable to use them when she needed them most. A "Rebellious" part would stubbornly refuse to engage.

Her therapist, using IFS, asked Sarah, "What is the Rebellious part trying to do when you try to use those skills?"

The Rebellious part revealed it felt stifled and controlled by the expectation to just "tolerate" pain. It feared that using skills meant suppressing its voice and that its pain would never be heard. Sarah's Self, with the therapist's guidance, acknowledged this: "I see you're worried about being silenced, and that's a fair concern." From this compassionate place, Sarah's Self negotiated with the Rebellious part, suggesting that using a skill was not about silencing, but about creating enough space for the Self to eventually hear and help the deeper pain. The Rebellious part, feeling respected, agreed to allow Sarah to use skills as a temporary measure, knowing her Self would eventually listen to its message. This shifted from mere behavioral compliance to internal cooperation.

Case Example 2: IFS-Informed Emotion Regulation for Overwhelmed Firefighters

Mark often experienced intense anger outbursts, driven by a Firefighter part that reacted to perceived slights. While DBT taught him emotion regulation skills like "opposite action," he found it hard to apply them in the heat of the moment.

His therapist helped Mark's Self connect with the Angry Firefighter. "Angry part, what are you so upset about? What are you protecting?" The Firefighter revealed a profound sense of injustice and a fear that Mark would be taken advantage of if he did not react forcefully, protecting a "Vulnerable" Exile. Instead of just applying opposite action (which the Firefighter resisted), Mark's Self first offered compassion to the Firefighter, validating its protective intent. "I see you're fighting to protect me from being hurt again." Then, Mark's Self, with the Firefighter's permission, applied an emotion regulation skill, but with a different intention: not to suppress the anger, but to create enough calm for the Self to address the vulnerable Exile underneath. This IFS-informed application made the DBT skill feel less like a rigid rule and more like a compassionate tool for internal care.

Case Example 3: Transforming the Self-Critic with IFS, not Just Challenging It

Lisa suffered from severe self-criticism, constantly belittling herself and undermining her achievements. DBT taught her to challenge these negative thoughts. While helpful, the thoughts often returned with force.

Her therapist used IFS to invite Lisa's Self to dialogue with the Self-Critic part. "Self-Critic, I hear how harsh you are. What are you afraid would happen if you were kind to Lisa?" The Self-Critic, surprisingly, revealed its deep fear that Lisa would become lazy or incompetent if it stopped pushing her. It was a Manager part, trying to protect an Exile that felt inherently flawed. Lisa's Self listened with compassion, acknowledging the Self-Critic's protective intent. "I see you're trying to help me be better, and I appreciate that. But your harshness actually hurts me." Lisa's Self then offered to take on the responsibility of guiding her towards her goals with kindness, assuring the Self-Critic that it did not need to be so harsh. This approach transformed the Self-Critic, allowing it to soften its voice and become an inner cheerleader rather than a tormentor, which was much more lasting than simply challenging the thoughts.

Neurofeedback

Neurofeedback is a method that uses real-time displays of brain activity to teach people how to control their own brain function [41, 42]. While we are still learning about how to directly combine it with IFS, the benefits of neurofeedback can really help IFS work by:

- **Calming the Nervous System:** Neurofeedback can help calm the nervous system, reducing things like anxiety, sadness, and feeling too revved up—all common with complex trauma [41, 42]. When the nervous system is calmer, it creates a more stable inner environment. This makes it easier for people to connect with their Self and work with their parts without getting overwhelmed [41].

- **Improving Self-Awareness:** By showing you what your brain is doing in the moment, neurofeedback can help you become more aware of your inner states [41]. This can support the IFS process of spotting and telling apart your different parts [41].

- **Better Emotional Regulation:** As people learn to control their brain activity, they might find they are better at managing their emotions [41]. This can reduce the need for extreme protective behaviors and help with deeper IFS work [41].

Let us look at some examples:

Case Example 1: Reducing Hyper-Vigilance for Easier IFS Access

Mark, a client with CPTSD, struggled to access his inner parts because of extreme hyper-vigilance. His brain activity showed consistent high beta waves (associated with alertness and anxiety), making him feel constantly on edge.

His therapist began integrating neurofeedback sessions alongside IFS. The neurofeedback trained Mark's brain to produce more alpha waves (associated with calm and relaxation) and less high beta. As his nervous system became more regulated through neurofeedback, Mark reported feeling less jumpy and more grounded. This allowed him to more easily access his Self during IFS sessions and engage with his frightened protectors without them feeling overwhelmed or needing to shut down, thereby accelerating the IFS unburdening work.

Case Example 2: Enhancing Awareness of Parts' States

Sarah found it hard to tell if she was blended with a part or in Self, especially when her "Anxious" part took over. Her brain patterns would show specific activity when this part was dominant.

Her therapist used neurofeedback to help Sarah visually see her brain activity. When her "Anxious" part was active, a specific brain wave pattern would appear on the screen. The therapist would then ask, "What part is active right now?" Sarah learned to connect the visual feedback with her internal experience. This real-time feedback helped her quickly identify when she was blended with the Anxious part versus when she was in her Self. This enhanced awareness made her much more skilled at unblending and leading from her Self during IFS sessions.

Case Example 3: Stabilizing Mood for Deeper Trauma Processing

David experienced severe mood swings and periods of deep despair, which were Firefighter responses to a deeply buried Exile holding shame. His emotional dysregulation made consistent IFS work challenging.

His therapist integrated neurofeedback to help stabilize David's mood. By training his brain to regulate specific emotional circuits, the neurofeedback helped reduce the intensity and frequency of his mood swings. As David's emotional system became more stable, his Self was able to stay present for longer periods. This reduced the Firefighter's need to jump in with extreme responses, creating a more consistent and safe internal environment. This stability allowed for much deeper and more sustained work in IFS sessions, where David's Self could finally access and unburden the shame held by his Exile without becoming overwhelmed by intense mood shifts.

Psychedelic-Assisted Therapy

The meeting point of IFS and **psychedelic-assisted therapy** is getting a lot of attention because it can bring about really deep healing [43, 44]. IFS is a natural fit for this kind of therapy because it does not label things as wrong and focuses on what is happening inside a person [43].

Here is why IFS works so well with psychedelic-assisted therapy:

- **Preparation and Integration:** IFS gives you a strong way to get ready for psychedelic experiences and to help you make sense of the new understandings you gain during sessions [43, 44]. Psychedelics can make hidden thoughts and feelings much stronger, bringing deep patterns, traumas, and inner struggles into your conscious mind [43].

- **Handling Intense Experiences:** By using the IFS view, people can work with their inner dynamics in a structured and supportive way during psychedelic sessions [43, 44]. This helps them be curious and kind towards their inner parts (like a wounded child, an inner critic, or a protector) instead of feeling completely overwhelmed [43].

- **Self-Led Presence:** IFS encourages people to bring their compassionate and curious Self into their psychedelic experiences [43, 44]. This provides a steady and nurturing presence even when things feel chaotic inside [43]. This builds safety and trust within themselves, leading to lasting change and helping them bring their new understandings into their daily life [43].

Let us look at some examples:

Case Example 1: IFS Preparation for Psilocybin Session

Sarah was preparing for a psilocybin-assisted therapy session to address long-standing trauma. She had a "Terrified Child" Exile and a "Control" Manager that feared losing control during the psychedelic experience.

Her therapist used IFS *before* the session to help Sarah's Self connect with the Control Manager. "Control part, I see you're worried about what might happen during the session. What are you afraid of?" The Manager expressed its fear of chaos and overwhelming emotions. Sarah's Self, guided by the therapist, reassured the Manager that the Self would remain present as an anchor and that they would go at the pace the system needed. They also developed a clear intention for the session, focusing on the Self's desire to meet the Terrified Child with compassion. This IFS preparation helped the Control Manager relax its grip, allowing Sarah to approach the psychedelic experience with less anxiety and more openness, knowing her Self was ready to lead.

Case Example 2: Navigating a Challenging Psilocybin Experience with IFS

During a psychedelic session, Mark encountered intense anger and rage, seemingly from a "Rage" Firefighter part that he had rarely accessed before. He felt overwhelmed and wanted to shut it down.

His therapist, trained in IFS, gently reminded Mark to bring his Self to the experience. "Mark, can your Self turn towards that anger? What is the Rage part trying to tell you?" Mark's Self, through the guidance, was able to view the Rage not as a threat, but as a part with a message. The Rage part showed him images of past injustices where he felt utterly powerless. Instead of fighting the anger, Mark's Self, with the therapist's support, allowed the Rage to be fully felt, compassionately witnessing its intensity. This IFS lens allowed Mark to move through the experience with curiosity rather than fear, leading to a profound understanding and eventual softening of the Rage part, freeing an Exile carrying deep feelings of powerlessness.

Case Example 3: IFS Integration of Psychedelic Insights

Lisa had a profound psychedelic experience where she saw a "burden" of shame, passed down from her ancestors, as a heavy cloak she was wearing. She felt immense relief but was unsure how to make this insight last.

Her therapist used IFS *after* the psychedelic session for integration. They helped Lisa's Self connect with the "Shame-Wearing" part she had seen. Lisa's Self asked the part, "Now that you've seen this cloak, are you ready to take it off?" Lisa, from her Self, visualized gently removing the heavy cloak and placing it in a sacred space, no longer needing to carry it. They then discussed how this shift could impact her daily life, identifying what Manager parts might try to re-impose the shame, and how her Self could lead in those moments. This IFS integration helped Lisa translate the powerful psychedelic insight into a lasting internal shift, embodying the unburdening in a practical way.

Concluding Thoughts

The journey into advanced IFS shows us that healing is not always a straight line. It is a dance between understanding, compassion, and skilled intervention. By embracing the flexibility of IFS and combining it with other powerful modalities, we can help people find deeper levels of freedom and wholeness than ever before. This truly is the art of helping people come home to themselves.

Key Learnings

- **IFS for CPTSD:** See extreme symptoms as protectors. Engage them directly, help regulate the nervous system, witness and unburden pain, and restore Self-leadership.

- **IFS for DID:** Approach alters as protective parts, not pathologies. Foster communication among them through the core Self, promoting harmony and integration by creating a safe inner space.

- **IFS and EMDR:** Use IFS to build safety, identify trauma-holding parts, reduce resistance, and deepen processing within EMDR sessions.

- **IFS and Somatic Approaches:** Combine IFS with SE and Polyvagal Theory to address bodily stored trauma. Increase body awareness, regulate the nervous system, embody Self-energy, and process implicit memories for physiological unburdening.

- **IFS and DBT:** IFS heals the root pain that makes DBT skills hard to use. It helps parts accept skills, transforms self-criticism, and addresses resistance to skills for lasting change.

- **IFS and Neurofeedback:** Neurofeedback helps regulate the nervous system, making it easier to access Self and parts. It also enhances self-awareness and emotional regulation for deeper IFS work.

- **IFS and Psychedelic Therapy:** IFS offers a framework for preparing for and integrating psychedelic experiences, navigating intense internal dynamics, and maintaining a Self-led presence for lasting transformation.

Helping folks untangle their inner knots can be tricky business. Imagine working with someone whose own mind seems to fight them every step of the way. You might call that "resistance," but what if we saw it not as a battle, but as a silent plea from parts of them trying to keep things safe? This way of thinking — seeing those inner struggles as protectors doing their very best, even when it looks like they're holding things back — changes everything. It opens the door to a kinder, more effective way of helping, one where we befriend those protective walls instead of trying to tear them down.

Chapter 6: Getting Through Tricky Client Situations

Handling Resistance: Befriending Inner Protectors

You see, what we often label as "resistance" in therapy isn't really someone trying to be difficult or defy your suggestions. Not at all! It's simply the hard work of inner **parts** trying to keep the person from what they fear most. These parts, bless their hearts, truly believe they're preventing more hurt or overwhelming feelings. Think of them as diligent, if sometimes misguided, guardians.

When someone shows "resistance," it simply means their protectors are standing tall, doing their job. Our job as therapists? To understand their mission, not to fight it. We're not looking to dismantle these protectors; we're looking to understand what they're so worried about. This changes everything from an adversarial dance to a curious exploration.

Here are some good ways to work with those protective parts:

- **Respecting the Protector's Good Aim:** Always approach a part that seems to be resisting with true respect and a sense of wonder. Acknowledge its positive goal, even if its ways seem to gum up the works. This act of acknowledging what the part is trying to do — even if it's clumsy — helps it feel seen and understood. When a part feels seen, it doesn't need to shout so loudly or put up such a strong front. It's like saying, "Hey, I get that you're trying to help, and I appreciate that."

- - **Case Example 6.1:** Sarah, a client, consistently missed appointments or showed up late, making excuses that seemed flimsy. Instead of getting frustrated, her therapist, Dr. Chen, asked, "Sarah, a part of you seems to be making it hard to get here on time. What might that part be trying to protect you from by keeping you from our sessions?" Sarah paused, then admitted, "It's like a part of me is afraid that if I really get into this, I'll have to face how angry I am, and then I'll just fall apart." Dr. Chen responded, "That part is doing a good job trying to keep you from falling apart. It sounds like it's trying to protect you from something really big." This acknowledgment helped Sarah's "late" part relax a bit, seeing that Dr. Chen wasn't going to force her to "fall apart."

- **Knowing Their Fears:** You simply must find out what these resistant parts are truly scared of. Ask questions like, "**What are you afraid would happen if you relaxed this protection?**" or "**What's the worst-case scenario this part is trying to prevent?**" This sort of inquiry, coming from your own **Self-energy**, builds trust. When a part feels like it's truly being heard, it often becomes less rigid. It's not about arguing with the part; it's about listening to its story.

  - **Case Example 6.2:** Mark was having trouble talking about his childhood experiences. Every time the conversation got close, he'd change the subject or crack a joke. His therapist, Lisa, noticed this pattern. One day, she gently asked, "There's a part of you, Mark, that seems to pull you away when we get close to talking about your past. What is that part worried would happen if you really spoke about those things?" Mark shifted uncomfortably, then said, "It thinks I'll just get swallowed by it, that I'll never stop crying, or I'll just explode." Lisa replied, "So this part is trying to keep you from being overwhelmed, from feeling too much. That's a very good reason for it to act the way it does." By helping Mark name the fear, his protective part felt understood, and he was able to share a little more about what it was holding back.

- **Letting the Client Guide:** Make it absolutely clear that the client is "**fully in the driver's seat**." Nothing will happen without their clear permission and the agreement of their parts. This respects their **autonomy** and helps those protective parts feel less like they need to be in absolute control. When a part knows it has a say, it often doesn't need to fight so hard for its position. We're not here to take over; we're here to offer a different path.

    - **Case Example 6.3:** David had a part that would shut down his feelings completely when his wife brought up any conflict. His therapist, Dr. Lee, noticed this blank look. "David," she said, "a part of you goes completely still when things get heated. We can work with that part, but only when it feels completely safe, and only if it agrees. You are in charge of how fast we go and what we do." David's face softened a little. "You mean I don't have to push through it?" Dr. Lee nodded. "Exactly. We'll listen to what that part needs to feel safe before we do anything else." This reassurance gave David's protective part a sense of control, making it more willing to allow exploration.

- **Showing What's to Gain:** Gently talk about the good things that might happen for the resistant part if it could just ease up a bit. For example, it wouldn't have to work so hard! Protectors use up a lot of **energy** keeping things bottled up. Imagine the relief they might feel if they didn't have to carry such a heavy load. It's about painting a picture of a lighter, freer existence for them.

- **Confirming the Pain and Hope:** Acknowledge that what the client is going through right now hurts. And yes, the healing process might bring up some uncomfortable feelings. But always, always hold out **hope for change**. It's okay to say, "I see your pain, and I know this might be tough, but I truly believe things can get better." This balance—acknowledging the difficulty while keeping a vision of betterment—can be very comforting.

This way of looking at resistance flips the script. It's not a block to therapy; it's a window into the client's inner workings. It gives us vital clues about their protective plans and allows for a deeper, more profound kind of healing.

Working with Extreme Parts: Suicidality and Self-Harm

When folks are dealing with really tough stuff, like thoughts of ending their life or self-harm, it calls for a very steady and

Self-led approach. We always, always put the client's **safety** first. But even with these serious situations, we still use the same understanding of inner parts.

Here are some ways to help when these extreme protectors show up:

- **Seeing Suicidal Thoughts Differently:** Don't think of suicidal thoughts or self-harm as something "wrong" with the person. Instead, see them as extreme efforts by protective parts—often those **Firefighters** we've talked about—to deal with pain that feels too much to bear. These parts are trying desperately to escape overwhelming hurt or a feeling of no way out. This way of seeing things lets you connect with compassion, rather than trying to shut them down right away. It's about asking, "What is this part trying to do *for* you?" not "What's wrong with you for thinking that?"

- **Finding the Good Intention:** Talk directly with the parts that are holding onto suicidal thoughts or urges to self-harm. Try to get their story, to really understand what good thing they're trying to achieve. Maybe they're trying to stop awful pain, or to feel *something* when everything feels numb, or to gain some control when life feels out of control. Ask questions like, "**What are you trying to accomplish by thinking about this?**" or "**What are you afraid would happen if you didn't do this?**" These questions are super important.

    - **Case Example 6.4:** Sarah, a 19-year-old, came to therapy reporting urges to cut herself when overwhelmed. Her therapist, Michael, rather than focusing solely on stopping the behavior, asked, "Sarah, there's a part of you that wants to cut. What is that part trying to do for you? What's its goal?" Sarah, tearfully, said, "It's trying to make me feel something other than just... nothing. And sometimes, it makes the big feelings inside go away for a little while." Michael responded, "So this part is trying to help you manage overwhelming emotions and feel less numb. That's a powerful job it's doing." By acknowledging the part's positive intent, Sarah felt understood, and the cutting part was less likely to feel attacked and more willing to communicate.

- **Talking It Over and Finding New Paths:** From a place of calm and clear **Self-energy**, you can talk with these parts. Offer them other ways to ease the pain. Give them a glimmer of **hope** that healing is truly possible. Ask them if they'd be willing to step back, even for a short time, to let other parts or your client's own **Self** find different answers. It's like saying, "I know you're trying to help, but are you open to letting us try a different approach?"

    o **Case Example 6.5:** David, who struggled with intense suicidal ideation, was working with his therapist, Emily. His suicidal part was very strong, convinced it was the only way out of his suffering. Emily spoke to this part directly, saying, "I hear you, part of David, and I see how much pain you're trying to end. It seems like you truly believe this is the only way to help David feel better. Are you willing to just step back a little, even for a few hours, to see if

David's Self and I can find a tiny bit of relief for him in another way?" Surprisingly, the part agreed to a temporary stepping back, allowing David to experience a moment of calm and hope, which hadn't been possible before.

- **Sharing Your Self-Energy:** When your client is really scared or feels completely hopeless, you might need to "**lend Self-energy**" to their system. This means you stay a steady, **compassionate** presence that their parts can lean on. This helps soften any arguments between their parts and creates room for their own **Self** to show up. Your calm, caring presence can be a lifeline.

- **Getting to the Root of the Pain:** The big goal here is to help those deeply wounded parts—the **Exiles**—that these extreme protectors are working so hard to hide. When those Exiles heal, there's no longer a need for such drastic measures. It's like finding and fixing the real problem, so the alarm bells don't have to ring anymore.

- **Knowing Your Own Stuff:** As a therapist, you must be really clear about your own inner parts that might get stirred up by a client talking about suicide or self-harm. You might have parts that feel afraid, or parts that want to jump in and "rescue." It's so important to "**unblend**" from these inner reactions. This helps you stay calm and clear, coming from your **Self**. If you're blended with your own fear, you might accidentally make your client's extreme part think it's the only solution.

Key Takeaways

- "Resistance" isn't defiance; it's a protector's job to prevent feared outcomes.
- Approaching protective parts with respect and curiosity about their fears can soften their stance.
- Always let the client know they are in control of the pace and depth of the work.
- Extreme parts like those involved in suicidality and self-harm are also trying to protect, often from unbearable pain.
- Talk directly to these parts, understand their positive intentions, and negotiate for alternative ways to find relief.
- Your steady, compassionate presence (lending Self-energy) can help calm a client's system.
- Remember that the ultimate aim is to heal the underlying wounded parts.
- Therapists must be aware of their own inner reactions to challenging client material and work from their own **Self-energy**.

Chapter 7: Ethics and Growing as a Professional

Working with people in such a deep way, especially with complex situations, brings up some important questions about what's right and what's fair. It also means we, as therapists, have to keep learning and growing, and just as important, take really good care of ourselves.

Hard Ethical Choices: Power and Limits

In therapy, there's always a power difference. You, the therapist, are the guide, and the client is often in a very open, vulnerable place. With how deeply we work in IFS, this difference becomes even clearer. We step into the client's inner world, which is a very private space indeed.

Here are some important ethical ideas to keep close:

- **Client's Freedom and Doing Good:** We must always uphold a client's right to choose for themselves, even if their choices make us worried. At the same time, we need to always act in their best interest. This means we have to really check if someone can make clear decisions, especially if they have developmental delays or severe mental illness. As therapists, we should avoid telling people what to do. Our aim is to help the client's **Self** grow strong enough to make their own good choices.
    - **Case Example 7.1:** A client, Maria, with a history of severe anxiety, suddenly decided she wanted to stop taking her prescribed medication, which had been helping stabilize her. Her therapist, Dr. Rodriguez, felt a strong

urge to tell her she was making a bad decision. However, remembering the principle of client **autonomy**, Dr. Rodriguez instead asked Maria, "A part of you wants to stop taking your medication. What is that part hoping will happen? What are its concerns about staying on it?" They discussed the potential risks and benefits, exploring Maria's parts that desired more independence and those that feared medication. Dr. Rodriguez helped Maria make an informed choice, respecting her decision while ensuring she understood the possible outcomes, rather than simply telling her what to do.

- **Double Relationships and Clear Lines:** You must recognize and strictly avoid having any kind of **dual relationship** with a client. This means no accepting personal favors, no asking for testimonials, and definitely no personal friendships. These things can mess up the power balance and hurt the therapeutic bond. Even something that seems innocent can break **confidentiality** or take advantage of a client's vulnerability. Keep those boundaries clear and strong.

- **Keeping Secrets:** You must keep client information private. This is a strict rule. You also need to understand when you *have* to share information, for example, if someone is in danger, or if the law requires it. Always be clear with your clients about these limits.

- **Knowing What You Can Do and When You Need Help:** Therapists have a moral duty to work only within what they are truly good at. This means you need to know your limits. You also have to deal with anything in your own life—like feeling burned out or letting your own feelings get in the way—that might keep you from doing your best work. If you're not doing well, you can't help others as well as you should.

Your Own Inner World and How It Affects Therapy

Just like our clients, we therapists have our own inner systems of parts. And believe me, these parts will always, always show up in the therapy room! When we talk about **countertransference**, we're simply talking about our own inner reactions to our clients. It's a natural thing; it's going to happen.

Advanced IFS therapy really pushes us to do this:

- **Knowing Your Own Therapist Parts:** You've got to work on truly understanding your own inner landscape. Notice your own **Managers**, **Firefighters**, and **Exiles** that get stirred up by what clients bring in. This means spotting your "therapist parts"—those parts of you that want to fix everything, or rescue everyone, or might even feel overwhelmed. If these parts take over, they can actually hurt your clients.

- **Stepping Back from Countertransference:** Learn ways to "**unblend**" from those activated therapist parts when you feel your own reactions bubbling up. This lets you respond from your own **Self-energy**, keeping your boundaries steady and staying effective. It also stops you from misunderstanding your client or crossing ethical lines. It's about noticing, "Oh, that's *my* fear showing up," rather than believing it's the client's.

- **Using Countertransference as a Clue:** Don't see your own reactions as a problem to get rid of. Instead, think of them as useful information about your client's inner world and their ways of relating. For example, if you feel a super strong urge to "save" a client, it might be a signal that there's a client part that is trying to get you to play that rescuer role. It's a message from their system to yours.

- **Getting Help and Talking Things Over:** Regular talks with other therapists and supervisors are so important. This is how you figure out those complicated countertransference moments and make sure you're always working ethically, especially when cases get tough. You don't have to figure it all out alone.

Taking Care of Yourself and Avoiding Burnout

Working with deep hurt and highly defended inner systems can be really draining. It can even lead to you feeling traumatized yourself, or totally burned out. Taking care of yourself isn't just a nice thing to do; it's a requirement for being a good therapist over the long haul.

Here are some ways to keep yourself steady, using what we know from IFS:

- **Being Aware of Your Own Parts:** Keep checking in with your own inner world. How might your own parts be shaping how you respond to your clients? This stops you from accidentally putting your own stuff onto your clients or reacting in ways that don't help them heal.

- **Kindness to Self and Leading Your Own System:** Apply the same IFS principles to yourself! Be **compassionate** with your own parts. Lead your own system from your **Self**. This builds up your inner strength and helps you deal with stress so you don't burn out. You can't pour from an empty cup, as they say.

- **Setting Your Limits:** Know your personal limits in your professional work. Learn to say "no" when you need to, and clearly tell others what you need. This means managing how many clients you see and making sure you get enough rest and personal time. Your time and energy are precious resources.

- **Keeping on Growing:** Keep learning and making the IFS model a part of your own life. This might mean getting your own therapy, doing meditations, or trying out the exercises yourself. The more you truly live the IFS way, the better you'll be at helping others do the same.

- **Support from Others:** Connect with other IFS therapists. Share what you're learning, ask for their advice, and support each other. This helps you avoid feeling alone and gives you a place to talk through tough experiences. We're all in this together.

What to Hold Onto

- Always respect client **autonomy** while also acting in their best interest, especially with tricky ethical choices.

- Strictly avoid **dual relationships** to maintain clear **boundaries** and protect the therapeutic connection.

- **Confidentiality** is paramount, with clear understanding of its limits.

- Therapists must know their own limitations and address anything that could impair their work.

- Your own internal system influences therapy, so **self-awareness** of your "therapist parts" is key.

- Use **countertransference** as a source of information about the client's system, and learn to **unblend** from your own reactions.

- Regular **supervision** and consultation are essential for navigating complex dynamics.

- **Self-care** is not a luxury; it's an **ethical** necessity to prevent burnout and maintain effectiveness.

- Applying IFS principles to your own life—**self-compassion**, **self-leadership**, and setting **boundaries**—builds resilience.

- Connect with a **community** of practitioners for support and shared learning.

Reflections on the Path

As we consider the vast and often mysterious inner worlds of those we seek to help, it becomes abundantly clear that our work is never truly done. It is a continuous dance of discovery—of ourselves, of our clients, and of the incredible power within each human system to heal. The true art lies not in wielding some magical cure, but in creating a space where the inherent wisdom of the **Self** can emerge, guiding both client and therapist toward a deeper sense of wholeness and peace. It asks us to be brave enough to look inward, compassionate enough to hold another's pain, and humble enough to know we are always, always learning. It's a demanding path, to be sure, but one that offers profound rewards, for them and for us.

Chapter 8: The Current State of Research and New Directions

IFS is getting more and more attention as a therapy backed by good evidence. A growing amount of research shows it helps with many different problems.

What the Research Shows: Evidence and What We Still Need to Learn

IFS is becoming known as a therapy that works, and studies are showing its power across many situations.

- **Trauma — Including PTSD and CPTSD:** Early studies show IFS really helps reduce symptoms tied to trauma, especially from childhood. Research points to IFS making a big difference in how much people suffer from symptoms, and it helps them feel more self-compassion, handle emotions better, and see themselves in a more positive light after trauma [1].
    - Case Example 8.1: Maria's Journey with Childhood Trauma

Maria, a 40-year-old woman, came to therapy with a long history of feeling disconnected and easily overwhelmed. She often felt a strong inner critic — a part that constantly told her she wasn't good enough and that everything was her fault. She had nightmares and flashbacks to an abusive childhood. In IFS therapy, Maria began to meet these parts. She discovered her inner critic was trying to protect her from more pain, even though it was harsh. She also connected with a young, frightened part of herself that held the memories of the abuse. Through Self-led compassion and understanding, Maria was able to offer comfort to this young part. Over several months, her flashbacks lessened, and the critical voice softened. She felt more connected to herself and calmer, able to manage tough emotions without feeling completely lost. The healing from her childhood wounds truly began to take hold, showing how IFS helps untangle the knots of past hurts.

- **Feeling Down and Anxious:** Studies have shown IFS helps lessen feelings of sadness and worry. It guides people to build kinder relationships with their inner selves and feel less controlled by worried inner parts [2].
    - Case Example 8.2: David and His Anxious Parts

David, a 30-year-old software engineer, struggled with constant worry about his performance at work and in relationships. He often felt a churning in his stomach and a racing heart. He described a "what-if" part that always anticipated the worst. In IFS, David learned to approach this anxious part with curiosity. He discovered it was trying to keep him safe by preparing him for every possible bad outcome, even though it exhausted him. As David, from his Self, listened to this part and offered it reassurance, the intensity of his anxiety began to drop. He started noticing moments of peace he hadn't felt in years. He also found a playful part that had been hidden by his worry. By recognizing and appreciating these different parts, David gained more control over his anxiety and felt more balanced.

- **Addictions:** IFS has been good at helping with substance use problems. It does this by getting to the main reasons for the addiction, helping wounded inner parts, and calming inner conflicts [3].

- - Case Example 8.3: Sarah's Path to Freedom from Addiction

Sarah, a 45-year-old artist, found herself relying on alcohol to cope with stress and loneliness. She felt ashamed of her drinking and often tried to stop, only to find herself back in the same pattern. In IFS, Sarah identified a part of her that sought comfort and escape through alcohol, which she called her "comfort-seeker." She also found a deeply lonely and shamed part that the alcohol-seeking part was trying to protect. As Sarah connected with her Self, she was able to approach her comfort-seeker with understanding, rather than judgment. She also provided warmth and acceptance to her lonely part. This process allowed the comfort-seeker to relax its grip on alcohol, as the underlying needs were met in a healthier way. Sarah found new ways to cope with stress and began attending art classes again, truly changing her relationship with herself and with alcohol.

- **Dissociation and Related Conditions:** IFS is a powerful, evidence-based therapy used to treat dissociative problems, even Dissociative Identity Disorder (DID) [4].
  - Case Example 8.4: Mark and His Disconnected Selves

Mark, a 28-year-old student, often experienced gaps in his memory and a feeling of being detached from his own body. He had difficulty maintaining consistent relationships and often felt like different people at different times. Diagnosed with Dissociative Identity Disorder, Mark entered IFS therapy cautiously. Over time, he learned to identify and communicate with the various parts of his system, some of which held traumatic memories and others that served to protect him by dissociating. From his Self, Mark offered a calm, steady presence to his overwhelmed parts. He began to understand the roles each part played and how they were all trying to help him survive. This steady work helped Mark's system to become more integrated, reducing the memory gaps and increasing his sense of being a whole person. He started to feel more in control of his life and his experiences.

Despite these hopeful findings, there are still some missing pieces in the research:

- **Strong Research Needed:** While personal stories are powerful and early studies look good, we really need more big, careful research, including randomized controlled trials (RCTs). This would truly make IFS a widely accepted therapy that works for a broader set of conditions [5].

- **Severe Mental Health Issues:** We need to learn more about how well IFS works for very serious mental health problems, like schizophrenia and other complicated psychiatric conditions. Some people wonder if IFS alone can meet all the needs of these groups, suggesting they might need other therapies too [6].

- **Specific Uses:** There's a need for more research on how to create and test specific IFS-based treatment plans for particular problems, like excessive internet use [7].

- **Different Cultures:** More studies are needed to see how well IFS works and how it can be used in different cultures. We also need to learn how to change the approach to fit different cultural traditions and values [8].

New Directions in IFS Therapy

The field of IFS is seeing some exciting new directions that show us where it's going.

- **Putting IFS Together with Other Therapies:** People are looking more and more at how well IFS works with other therapies that are known to be effective. This includes combining it with EMDR (Eye Movement Desensitization and Reprocessing), Somatic Experiencing, Polyvagal Theory, and DBT (Dialectical Behavior Therapy). This creates more complete and effective ways to treat complicated trauma and trouble with managing emotions [9].
    - Case Example 8.5: Combining IFS and EMDR for Complex Trauma

Jessica, a 35-year-old, experienced severe anxiety and panic attacks stemming from years of emotional neglect in childhood. She felt overwhelmed by her emotions and often had vivid, distressing memories. Her therapist began with IFS, helping Jessica identify a frightened, young exile part holding the pain of neglect and a protector part that would send her into panic to keep her from feeling the neglect. Once Jessica, from her Self, could connect with and soothe these parts, the therapist introduced EMDR to process specific traumatic memories that the exile held. The combination allowed Jessica to unburden the emotional charge from the memories while also building a stronger connection with her inner parts. She reported feeling a significant reduction in panic attacks and a greater sense of inner calm, showing how these approaches can work hand-in-hand.

- **IFS and Psychedelic-Assisted Therapy:** IFS is becoming a top approach for preparing for and integrating experiences from psychedelic-assisted therapy. It uses its accepting view of inner parts to help people go through strong inner experiences and find deep healing [10].
    - Case Example 8.6: Using IFS for Psychedelic Integration

Tom, a 50-year-old man, underwent a therapist-guided psychedelic experience to address long-standing depression. During the session, he encountered intense feelings of unworthiness and saw visions of a shadowy figure representing his inner critic. Before the psychedelic session, his therapist used IFS to help Tom understand his internal system and how his inner critic functioned as a protector. After the session, IFS became the main framework for integration. Tom could approach the "shadowy figure" not as something to fear, but as a part of himself trying to help, albeit in a harsh way. He spent time with the feelings of unworthiness, allowing his Self to offer compassion to the parts that held those feelings. This IFS-guided integration helped Tom make sense of his psychedelic experience, leading to a lasting reduction in his depressive symptoms and a new sense of self-acceptance.

- **Focus on the Therapist's Inner System:** There's a growing understanding that a therapist's own inner system, how they react to clients (countertransference), and how they care for themselves are super important for good, ethical therapy. Training programs are adding more about how therapists can manage their own inner parts and handle countertransference [11].

- Case Example 8.7: Therapist Self-Awareness in Practice

Sarah, an experienced IFS therapist, found herself feeling unusually frustrated during sessions with a particular client, Michael, who seemed resistant to connecting with his vulnerable parts. Through her own personal IFS work and supervision, Sarah discovered she had a "fix-it" part that got frustrated when clients didn't make quick progress. She also realized Michael's resistance reminded her of her own struggles with vulnerability early in her career. By acknowledging and bringing her Self-energy to her "fix-it" part, Sarah was able to approach Michael with more patience and curiosity. This shift allowed Michael to feel safer, and he eventually began to open up, demonstrating how a therapist's internal work directly helps client progress.

- **Wider Uses:** Beyond traditional therapy, IFS is being explored in many areas like helping leaders develop, working with company teams, school management, and even in legal disagreements. This shows how flexible the model is for understanding human groups [12].

- **Bringing in Technology:** The creation of tools like the IFS Guide App suggests a future where technology might help with mapping inner parts, keeping track of inner conversations, and even simulating internal dialogues. This would support both clients and therapists in their work [13].

Key Takeaways

- IFS shows strong potential in helping with trauma, anxiety, sadness, addiction, and dissociation, with a growing research base.

- More rigorous research, including large-scale trials, is needed to solidify IFS as a widely accepted approach for a broader array of conditions.

- Research also needs to look at IFS's use in severe mental illnesses, specific problems like internet overuse, and its effectiveness across different cultures.

- New directions in IFS include combining it with other therapies (like EMDR and Polyvagal Theory), its use in psychedelic-assisted therapy, a focus on the therapist's own internal world, wider applications beyond therapy, and integrating technology.

Chapter 9: A Call for More Research and Professional Growth

To truly establish IFS as a leading, advanced way of doing therapy, we need more focused research.

What Research Still Needs to Explore

To make IFS even stronger as a top therapeutic method, certain areas need focused research:

- **Randomized Controlled Trials (RCTs):** We need more big, careful RCTs to give solid proof of how well IFS works for a wider range of complicated clinical issues, including serious mental health problems and specific personality conditions [14].

- **How IFS Works:** Studies that look into the exact ways IFS causes change – for example, how Self-leadership directly affects brain pathways, or how unburdening changes emotional regulation on a physical level – would help us understand and improve the techniques [15].

- **Long-Term Studies:** Research that tracks what happens long-term after IFS interventions in complicated cases is needed to see if the changes last and how well people avoid problems coming back [16].

- **Comparing Different Treatments:** We need to compare IFS, both by itself and when combined with other therapies, against other known treatments for complicated conditions. This will help us figure out the best ways to help people [17].

- **Adapting for Different Cultures:** Research on how to adjust IFS for different cultures is important. This makes sure it works well and can be used by people from all backgrounds and ways of seeing the world [18].
- **Therapist's Role:** Studies looking at how a therapist's Self-energy, how they manage their own reactions (countertransference), and their self-care practices affect how clients do in complicated cases are also crucial [19].

Continuing Professional Growth for Advanced IFS Therapists

The constantly changing nature of IFS and the challenging aspects of advanced clinical work make ongoing professional growth extremely important.

- **Advanced Training and Certification:** Getting involved in IFS Level 2 and Level 3 trainings is a smart move. These trainings really focus on the fine points, like working with tough shame, trauma from very early life, inner systems that are very divided, and telling the difference between true Self-energy and parts that just *seem* like Self [20].
- **Specialized Workshops and Classes:** Taking part in workshops that really dig into specific advanced techniques is a great idea. Think about things like Somatic IFS, combining with EMDR or DBT, or handling those particularly extreme inner parts [21].
- **Talking with Supervisors:** Regularly talking with experienced IFS supervisors is a must. This helps you handle tough cases, work through your own reactions

to clients (countertransference), and get better at your clinical abilities [22].

- **Personal IFS Work:** Doing your own therapy and exploring yourself using the IFS model is truly essential for therapists. This helps you get more in touch with your own Self, manage your own inner system, and avoid feeling completely worn out. When you truly live the model, it makes you a stronger and more effective presence in the therapy room [23].

- **Staying Current with Research:** Keeping up with the latest research findings is wise. Also, contributing to the growing body of evidence through your own clinical work, and, if you can, taking part in research projects, helps everyone [24].

A Concluding Reflection

Internal Family Systems therapy gives us a truly understanding and effective way to deal with the many layers of the human mind, especially when working with difficult situations in therapy. The way this model doesn't label inner parts as "sick," but instead sees all of them as having good intentions, completely changes how therapy feels. It allows for a deeper connection and real healing.

This discussion has looked at the deeper ideas behind IFS, like understanding the many parts of us, the strong nature of our Self, and the key difference between personal burdens and those passed down through generations. It has also gone into detail about advanced techniques. These include working with parts that are disconnected, helping "exiles" let go of their burdens, strengthening Self-leadership, mapping out the inner system, and sorting out inner conflicts. These techniques give therapists powerful tools to navigate the complex inner worlds of people dealing with severe trauma, dissociative issues, and stubborn addictions.

What's more, putting IFS together with other trusted therapies—like EMDR, Somatic Experiencing, Polyvagal Theory, DBT, Neurofeedback, and even psychedelic-assisted therapy—shows how flexible the model is. It can create truly powerful combined effects, offering complete and personalized paths to healing. The emphasis on the therapist's own inner world, managing their reactions, and making sure practice is ethical and includes self-care points to the serious demands and responsibilities of advanced IFS work.

While IFS has shown promising results with many different groups of people in therapy, the need for more careful research remains important to make its evidence stronger and to see all it can do for the full range of complex mental health conditions. Ongoing professional growth, including advanced training, supervision, and personal IFS work, is essential for therapists to develop the Self-led presence and fine-tuned abilities needed to guide clients through their deepest healing journeys. Ultimately, IFS offers therapists a powerful and hopeful way forward, helping them bring about deep change and lasting inner calm, even in the most challenging situations.

References

[1] Schwartz, R. C. (1993). *Internal Family Systems Therapy*. Guilford Press.

[2] IFS Institute. (n.d.). *What is Internal Family Systems?* Retrieved from https://ifs-institute.com/

[3] GoodTherapy. (n.d.). *Internal Family Systems (IFS): Benefits, Techniques & How It Works*. Retrieved from https://www.goodtherapy.org/learn-about-therapy/types/internal-family-systems-therapy

[4] O'Connor de Boer, K. (2023). *Integrating Internal Family Systems Therapy into a phase-based approach for complex trauma*. Swinburne Research Bank. Retrieved from https://researchbank.swinburne.edu.au/file/83462f28-969e-4e9d-b338-46bb522c8641/1/kathleen_o_connor_de_boer_thesis.pdf

[5] Sage Leaf Wellness. (n.d.). *IFS and EMDR: A Powerful Combination for Healing Trauma*. Retrieved from https://www.sageleafwellness.com/blog/ifs-and-emdr-a-powerful-combination-of-healing-trauma

[6] Ava Recovery. (n.d.). *Internal Family Systems (IFS) Therapy for Addiction*. Retrieved from https://avarecovery.com/treatment/therapies/ifs/

[7] Therapy on Fig. (2024, October 11). *How IFS Can Help with Complex Trauma*. Retrieved from https://therapyonfig.com/blog/2024/10/11/how-ifs-can-help-with-complex-trauma

[8] eCare Behavioral Institute. (n.d.). *Treating Complex Trauma with Internal Family Systems*. Retrieved from

https://www.ecarebehavioralinstitute.com/courses/treating-complex-trauma-with-internal-family-systems/

[9] Internal Family Systems Portugal. (n.d.). *Four Types of Challenging Protectors with Chris Burris*. Retrieved from https://internalfamilysystems.pt/multimedia/webinars/four-types-challenging-protectors-chris-burris

[10] PESI UK. (n.d.). *Suicidality: An IFS Perspective*. Retrieved from https://www.pesi.co.uk/blogs/suicidality-an-ifs-perspective/

[11] IFS Telehealth Collective. (n.d.). *Dear Firefighter: What the IFS Model Can Offer to Those with Suicidal Thoughts*. Retrieved from https://ifstherapyonline.com/ifs-telehealth-collective-blog/dear-firefighter

[12] North Carolina State Bar. (n.d.). *Internal Family Systems as a Leadership Model*. Retrieved from https://www.ncbar.gov/for-lawyers/pathways-to-well-being/internal-family-systems-as-a-leadership-model/

[13] Celestial Twin. (n.d.). *IFS Self-Leadership - A Primer of Basic Concepts*. Retrieved from https://www.celestialtwin.com/ifs-self-leadership-a-primer-of-basic-concepts/

[14] Life Architect. (n.d.). *Self-energy and Self-like Parts in IFS | Workshop with Pamela Krause*. Retrieved from https://lifearchitect.com/self-energy-and-self-like-parts/

[15] Multiplicity of the Mind. (n.d.). *Inside the Therapist's Mind: Utilizing Internal Family Systems (IFS) to Navigate Countertransference*. Retrieved from https://multiplicityofthemind.com/therapists-have-parts-too-apr2025/

[16] IFS Healers. (n.d.). *Nuance and Attunement in the IFS Model*. Retrieved from https://www.ifshealers.com/c/nuance-and-attunement-in-the-ifs-model

[17] Casey Christian. (n.d.). *IFS Level 2 Training*. Retrieved from https://www.caseylpc.com/ifsintermediatetraining

[18] Crocker, T. C. (2023, May 21). *Becoming Whole: The Unburdening Process*. Medium. Retrieved from https://tomcrocker56.medium.com/becoming-whole-the-unburdening-process-2a913ec5e690

[19] EMDRIA. (n.d.). *EMDR Therapy and Internal Family Systems (IFS)*. Retrieved from https://www.emdria.org/blog/emdr-therapy-and-internal-family-systems-ifs/

[20] Sea Change Psychotherapy. (n.d.). *Dissociative Identity Disorder (DID)*. Retrieved from https://seachangepsychotherapy.com/services/dissociative-identity-disorder-did/

[21] MedCrave Online. (n.d.). *Dissociative Identity Disorder in the Context of Childhood Trauma and Anxiety: A Clinical Case Study Incorporating AI in Subconscious Energy Healing Therapy*. Retrieved from https://medcraveonline.com/JPCPY/dissociative-identity-disorder-in-the-context-of-childhood-trauma-and-anxiety-a-clinical-case-study-incorporating-ai-in-subconscious-energy-healing-therapy.html

[22] CareMe Health. (n.d.). *Internal Family Systems (IFS): Healing Parts of the Self*. Retrieved from https://careme.health/blog/internal-family-systems-ifs-healing-parts-of-the-self

[23] Tava Health. (n.d.). *Understanding Internal Family Systems (IFS) for Therapists*. Retrieved from https://www.tavahealth.com/blogs/internal-family-systems

[24] Lotus Center Therapy. (n.d.). *Let's Talk IFS Therapy*. Retrieved from https://lotuscentertherapy.com/lets-talk-ifs-therapy/

[25] Life Architect. (n.d.). *IFS Therapy & Complex Trauma - Workshop by Mike Elkin*. Retrieved from https://lifearchitect.com/ifs-therapy-complex-trauma-workshop-mike-elkin/

[26] Frontiers. (2022). *Case Report: Anomalous Experience in a Dissociative Identity and Borderline Personality Disorder*. Retrieved from https://www.frontiersin.org/journals/psychiatry/articles/10.3389/fpsyt.2022.662290/full

[27] ResearchGate. (n.d.). *Dissociative part-dependent biopsychosocial reactions to backward masked angry and neutral faces: An fMRI study of dissociative identity disorder*. Retrieved from https://www.researchgate.net/publication/258216540_Dissociative_part-dependent_biopsychosocial_reactions_to_backward_masked_angry_and_neutral_faces_An_fMRI_study_of_dissociative_identity_disorder

[28] Seattle Trauma Counseling. (n.d.). *Dissociative Identity Disorder (DID)*. Retrieved from https://seattletraumacounseling.com/services/dissociative-identity-disorder-did/

[29] Stroud Therapy. (n.d.). *Somatic IFS and polyvagal*. Retrieved from https://www.stroudtherapy.com/news/somaticifs

[30] Seattle Trauma Counseling. (n.d.). *Internal Family Systems*. Retrieved from https://www.seattletraumacounseling.com/specialties/internal-family-systems/

[31] The Encino Detox Center. (n.d.). *In-Depth Case Studies of the Internal Family Systems Model*. Retrieved from https://theencinodetoxcenter.com/in-depth-case-studies-of-the-internal-family-systems-model/

[32] NeuroColorado. (n.d.). *Healing from Complex Trauma*. Retrieved from https://www.neurocolorado.com/blog/healing-from-complex-trauma

[33] Kendhal Hart. (n.d.). *The Integrated EMDR and IFS Model Level 1*. Retrieved from https://www.kendhalhart.com/partstraining

[34] Stroud Therapy. (n.d.). *Somatic IFS and polyvagal*. Retrieved from https://www.stroudtherapy.com/news/somaticifs

[35] The Art of Embodiment. (n.d.). *Somatic Experiencing & Internal Family Systems - IFS*. Retrieved from https://www.artofembodiment.co.uk/about-2

[36] Life Architect. (n.d.). *IFS and the Polyvagal Theory. An online workshop with Alexia Rothman*. Retrieved from https://lifearchitect.com/ifs-and-the-polyvagal-theory/

[37] PESI. (n.d.). *Polyvagal-Informed, Internal Family Systems (IFS) Therapy: Healing Complex Trauma Through

Compassionate Connection. Retrieved from https://www.pesi.com/item/polyvagalinformed-internal-family-systems-ifs-therapy-healing-complex-trauma-compassionate-connection-152099

[38] IFS Guide. (n.d.). *Utilizing IFS Principles Alongside DBT Skills for Emotional Regulation and Interpersonal Effectiveness*. Retrieved from https://ifsguide.com/utilizing-ifs-principles-alongside-dbt-skills-for-emotional-regulation-and-interpersonal-effectiveness/

[39] IFS Guide. (n.d.). *Combining IFS and DBT*. Retrieved from https://ifsguide.com/combining-ifs-and-dbt/

[40] Reddit. (n.d.). *What are your (loving) critiques of IFS?*. Retrieved from https://www.reddit.com/r/InternalFamilySystems/comments/1ibgtuy/what_are_your_loving_critiques_of_ifs/

[41] Mendi.io. (n.d.). *fNIRS and EEG Neurofeedback: Combined Benefits for Mental Health*. Retrieved from https://www.mendi.io/blogs/brain-health/fnirs-and-eeg-neurofeedback-combined-benefits-for-enhanced-mental-health

[42] ISF Associates. (n.d.). *Neurofeedback Training & Educational Resources*. Retrieved from https://isfassociates.com/

[43] Transcendelic Retreats. (n.d.). *Exploring the Inner Landscape: Internal Family Systems and Psychedelic Therapy*. Retrieved from https://www.transcendelicretreats.com/blog/exploring-the-inner-landscape-internal-family-systems-and-psychedelic-therapy

[44] IFS with Sanni. (n.d.). *IFS for Psychedelic-Assisted Therapy Preparation & Integration*. Retrieved from https://www.ifswithsanni.com/psychedelic-assisted-therapy

[45] Private Practice Skills. (2025, January 13). *Dealing with Client Resistance: 4 Therapy Approaches*. Retrieved from https://privatepracticeskills.com/dealing-with-client-resistance-4-therapy-approaches/

[46] Internal Family Systems Portugal. (n.d.). *Four Types of Challenging Protectors with Chris Burris*. Retrieved from https://internalfamilysystems.pt/multimedia/webinars/four-types-challenging-protectors-chris-burris/

[47] IFS Telehealth Collective. (n.d.). *Dear Firefighter: What the IFS Model Can Offer to Those with Suicidal Thoughts*. Retrieved from https://ifstherapyonline.com/ifs-telehealth-collective-blog/dear-firefighter

[48] IFS Therapy Real Results. (n.d.). *FAQ*. Retrieved from https://www.ifstherapyrealresults.com/faq

[49] Johns Hopkins School of Nursing. (2018, February 27). *An Ethical Dilemma in Advanced Practice Nursing*. Retrieved from https://nursing.jhu.edu/magazine/articles/2018/02/ethical-dilemma-advanced-practice-nursing/

[50] IFS Institute. (n.d.). *Code of Conduct and Safety and Confidentiality Policy*. Retrieved from https://ifs-institute.com/resources/code-of-conduct

[51] Kasi Shan Therapy. (n.d.). *IFS Clinical Consultation*. Retrieved from https://kasishantherapy.com/ifs-consultation/

[52] PESI. (n.d.). *2-Day Advanced Workshop: Clinical Applications of Internal Family Systems (IFS) Therapy with Frank Anderson MD*. Retrieved from https://www.pesi.com/item/2day-advanced-workshop-clinical-applications-internal-family-systems-ifs-therapy-frank-anderson-md-57394

[53] Beyond Psychology Center. (n.d.). *Local Internal Family Systems (IFS) Therapy for Anxiety, Burnout, Trauma, Pain and Depression*. Retrieved from https://www.beyondpsychologycenter.com/internal-family-systems-therapy

[54] PESI. (n.d.). *Trauma Therapies Mastery*. Retrieved from https://www.pesi.com/sales/bh_c_002108_traumatherapiesmastery_organic-1010936

[55] Sea Change Psychotherapy. (n.d.). *Is Internal Family Systems (IFS) Evidence-Based?*. Retrieved from https://seachangepsychotherapy.com/posts/is-internal-family-systems-ifs-evidence-based/

[56] PTSD UK. (n.d.). *IFS research update*. Retrieved from https://www.ptsduk.org/ifs-research-update/

[57] Taylor & Francis Online. (n.d.). *The relationship between symptoms of complex posttraumatic disorder and core concepts in Internal Family Systems therapy*. Retrieved from https://www.tandfonline.com/doi/full/10.1080/13284207.2025.2467123

[58] ResearchGate. (n.d.). *Treating Complex Traumatic Stress Disorders / Internal Family Systems Therapy - Chapter 17*. Retrieved from https://www.researchgate.net/publication/327060001_Treat

ing_Complex_Traumatic_Stress_Disturbances_Internal_Family_Systems_Therapy_-_Chapter_17

[59] Swinburne Research Bank. (n.d.). *Integrating Internal Family Systems Therapy into a phase-based approach for complex trauma*. Retrieved from https://researchbank.swinburne.edu.au/file/83462f28-969e-4e9d-b338-46bb522c8641/1/kathleen_o_connor_de_boer_thesis.pdf

[60] ResearchGate. (n.d.). *Two Counselors Envision IFS (Internal Family Systems) Therapy for Addictions Treatment in Indian Country*. Retrieved from https://www.researchgate.net/publication/347197379_Two_Counselors_Envision_IFS_Internal_Family_Systems_Therapy_for_Addictions_Treatment_in_Indian_Country

[61] PMC. (n.d.). *A pilot study of an online group-based Internal Family Systems intervention for comorbid posttraumatic stress disorder and substance use*. Retrieved from https://pmc.ncbi.nlm.nih.gov/articles/PMC11983591/

[62] Good Woman Therapy. (n.d.). *IFS Therapy Criticism | Thoughts from an IFS Counselor in St. Louis, MO*. Retrieved from https://www.goodwomantherapy.com/blog/ifs-therapy-criticism-thoughts-from-an-ifs-counselor-st-louis-mo

[63] IFS Institute. (n.d.). *Research*. Retrieved from https://ifs-institute.com/resources/research

[64] Good Woman Therapy. (n.d.). *What are the problems with IFS Therapy? | Insights from an IFS Counselor*. Retrieved from https://www.goodwomantherapy.com/blog/what-are-the-problems-with-ifs

[65] PMC. (n.d.). *Development of an individual fitness score (IFS) based on the depression treatment guidelines of in the Japanese Society of Mood Disorders*. Retrieved from https://pmc.ncbi.nlm.nih.gov/articles/PMC10009429/

[66] Seattle Trauma Counseling. (n.d.). *Sensorimotor Psychotherapy*. Retrieved from https://www.seattletraumacounseling.com/specialties/sensorimotor-psychotherapy/

[67] Quarter Note Counseling. (n.d.). *Internal Family Systems (IFS)*. Retrieved from https://www.quarternotecounseling.com/internal-family-systems-ifs.html

[68] PESI. (n.d.). *Pat Ogden's Sensorimotor Psychotherapy for Complex Trauma*. Retrieved from https://www.pesi.com/sales/bh_c_001577_patogdencomplextrauma_organic-328416

[69] PESI. (n.d.). *Dissociation-Focused Trauma Treatment*. Retrieved from https://www.pesi.com/sales/bh_c_001571_dissociationfocusedtraumatreatment_organic-314820

[70] IFS Guide. (n.d.). *Advanced Techniques for Healing Trauma and Freeing Parts in IFS*. Retrieved from https://ifsguide.com/advanced-techniques-for-healing-trauma-and-freeing-parts-in-ifs/

[71] IFS Guide. (n.d.). *IFS Polarizations: Parts in Conflict*. Retrieved from https://ifsguide.com/ifs-polarizations-parts-in-conflict/

[72] The Encino Detox Center. (n.d.). *In-Depth Case Studies of the Internal Family Systems Model*. Retrieved from

https://theencinodetoxcenter.com/in-depth-case-studies-of-the-internal-family-systems-model/

[73] ResearchGate. (n.d.). *Two Counselors Envision IFS (Internal Family Systems) Therapy for Addictions Treatment in Indian Country*. Retrieved from https://www.researchgate.net/publication/347197379_Two_Counselors_Envision_IFS_Internal_Family_Systems_Therapy_for_Addictions_Treatment_in_Indian_Country

[74] IFS Telehealth Collective. (n.d.). *IFS Addiction Therapy*. Retrieved from https://ifstherapyonline.com/ifs-telehealth-collective-blog/ifs-addiction-therapy

[75] ERP Today. (n.d.). *When the Grid Gets Smart: TECO Energy's All-In Transformation with IFS*. Retrieved from https://erp.today/when-the-grid-gets-smart-teco-energys-all-in-erp-transformation-with-ifs/

[76] IFS. (n.d.). *Enterprise Resource Planning (ERP) Software Solutions*. Retrieved from https://www.ifs.com/solutions/enterprise-resource-planning/

[77] NBI Weston. (n.d.). *Complex Cases*. Retrieved from https://www.nbiweston.com/complex-cases

[78] Elsevier. (n.d.). *The relationship between clinical complexity and treatment outcome in psychotherapy: A systematic review*. Retrieved from https://www.elsevier.es/en-revista-european-journal-psychiatry-431-articulo-the-relationship-between-clinical-complexity-S0213616319301065

[79] University of Minnesota. (n.d.). *Case Study Involving Complex Trauma Part 3*. Retrieved from

https://cascw.umn.edu/case-study-involving-complex-trauma-part-3

[80] Sigma Marketplace. (n.d.). *Ethical Case Studies for Advanced Practice Nurses*. Retrieved from https://www.sigmamarketplace.org/ethical-case-studies-for-advance-practice-nurses

[81] BYU. (n.d.). *NURS 606 Advanced Practice Issues*. Retrieved from https://gradstudies.byu.edu/nurs-606-advanced-practice-issues

[82] PMC. (n.d.). *A Case Report of Complex Posttraumatic Stress Disorder with Paranoid and Histrionic Features Treated with Internal Family Systems Therapy*. Retrieved from https://pmc.ncbi.nlm.nih.gov/articles/PMC10837782/

www.ingramcontent.com/pod-product-compliance
Lightning Source LLC
Chambersburg PA
CBHW070303100426
42743CB00011B/2322